SpringerBriefs in Well-Being and
Quality of Life Research

For further volumes:
http://www.springer.com/series/10150

Bjørn Grinde

The Biology of Happiness

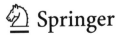 Springer

Bjørn Grinde
Division of Mental Health
Norwegian Institute of Public Health
PO Box 4404, Nydalen
0403 Oslo
Norway

ISSN 2211-7644
ISBN 978-94-007-4392-2
DOI 10.1007/978-94-007-4393-9
Springer Dordrecht Heidelberg New York London

e-ISSN 2211-7652
e-ISBN 978-94-007-4393-9

Library of Congress Control Number: 2012935720

Springer is part of Springer Science+Business Media (www.springer.com)

Preface

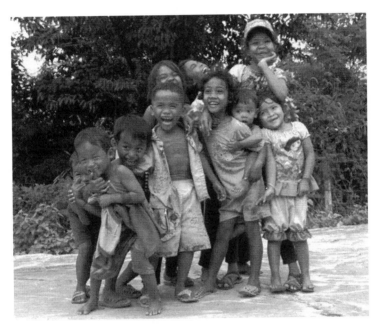

Cambodia is one of the poorest countries in the world, yet these children seem to have no problem finding happiness—perhaps because they have each other. The difficult part, however, is to retain happiness throughout life. (Photo: B. Grinde)

Happiness is a somewhat vague term. In the existing literature, most of it based on philosophy and the social sciences, it is possible to distinguish between two broad ways of applying the word. One is to use happiness as a value term for how life ought to be; i.e. somewhat synonymous with well-being, flourishing or quality of life. The other focuses on happiness as a particular emotional quality; i.e. pleasure as opposed to sorrow or pain. This split appears to date back to the early Greek literature, where they distinguished between eudaemonia (contentment and meaning) and hedonia (sensual pleasures).

I shall argue that the biological perspective on happiness unites the two alternatives in that it describes a common denominator for sensual pleasures, contentment, well being and flourishing. Although hedonia and eudaemonia are quite different as to how they are experienced, the affect part of both apparently has a shared evolutionary background, and is cared for by overlapping neural circuits.

The biologist Theodosius Dobzhansky once wrote, 'Nothing in biology makes sense except in the light of evolution'. More recently, the psychologist Henry Plotkin has suggested that in psychology nothing makes complete sense except in the light of evolution. The biological perspective has the power of creating an all-embracing platform for understanding human life, and thereby allowing for a unification of different approaches aimed at describing various topics—including the question of happiness.

In my mind, the purpose of science is to create the best possible model of reality. The aim of this book is to offer the best portrayal of what happiness is about, taking into consideration all the current evidence. Brain research is, however, a difficult subject; thus some of the details I add to my model are tentative. Even if it should be the best portrayal possible at the moment, which I am sure there are those who will dispute, it is unlikely to be so in 10 or 20 years.

Abstract

This book presents a model for what happiness is about—based on an evolutionary perspective. Briefly, the primary purpose of nervous systems is to direct an animal either towards opportunities or away from danger in order to help it survive and procreate. Three brain modules are engaged in this task: one for avoidance and two for attraction (seeking and consuming). While behaviour originally was based on reflexes, the brain gradually evolved into a more adaptive and flexible system based on positive and negative affects (good and bad feelings). The human capacity for happiness is presumably due to this whim of evolution—i.e. the advantages of having more flexibility in behavioural response. A variety of sub-modules have appeared, caring for a long list of pursuits, but recent studies suggest that they converge on shared neural circuits designed to generate positive and negative feelings. The brain functions involved in creating feelings, or affect, may collectively be referred to as mood modules. Happiness can be construed as the net output of these modules. Neural circuits tend to 'expand' (gain in strength and influence) upon frequent activation. This suggests the following strategy for improving mental health and enhancing happiness: To avoid excessive stimulation of negative modules, to use cognitive interference to enhance the 'turn off' function of these modules, and to exercise modules involved in positive feelings. In short, the evolutionary approach offers both a deeper understanding of happiness, and a framework for techniques aimed at improving well-being.

Contents

Chapter 1
Introduction: From Philosophy to Science

Abstract This chapter discusses what happiness is about, and whether 'happiness' can be used as a term for what should be the primary goal for both the individual and society. A historical look at thoughts about happiness is offered, as well as a discussion of the various terms used in this context. The chapter also covers an introduction to the evolutionary perspective of understanding the human mind.

Keywords Hedonism · Eudaimonia · Aristippus · Flourishing · Flow · Default contentment · Positive psychology · Darwinian happiness · Subjective wellbeing · Philosophy

1.1 Is Happiness What We Want?

The prospect of pleasure has been handed to us by the process of evolution. Evolution, however, aims towards survival and procreation; and happiness is biologically desirable only to the extent that it is relevant for these primary objectives. In other words, positive feelings evolved because they serve a purpose. Consequently, they are only available in species where this particular feature makes 'biological sense'—i.e. improves the survival of the genes. We happen to belong to one of these species. To take full advantage of the situation, we should understand what the capacity of happiness is about; just as we strive to understand other biological phenomena from the strategy of a viral infection to the functioning of a kidney.

It requires an advanced nervous system to experience any sort of feeling, which excludes all plants and most invertebrates. Your roses may flourish, and consequently make *you* happy, but the flowers themselves are incapable of sensations. Only animals that possess the right type of brain are able to enjoy life. (It presumably includes all mammals and to some extent birds and reptiles.). They have this capacity not because evolution is good hearted, but simply because feelings proved to be a useful evolutionary strategy.

B. Grinde, *The Biology of Happiness*, SpringerBriefs in Well-Being and Quality of Life Research, DOI: 10.1007/978-94-007-4393-9_1, © The Author(s) 2012

A variety of animals may be happy, but only one species—*Homo sapiens*—is in a position to understand what happiness is about, and thereby have some level of personal control over the situation. In other words, we can improve our quality of life not just beyond what is possible for other animals, but beyond the 'intentions' of the process that shaped our brains. Although happiness is an incidental by product of evolution; given this opportunity, should we not focus on how to make our allocated time on Earth as pleasant as possible?

There is a surprising variety of responses to this question.

Our distant ancestors were probably concerned about how to best enjoy life ever since they evolved the capacity for self-awareness and advanced cognition. Happiness is, arguably, the most important issue in life. As soon as our intellect allowed us to take advantage of our emotional brain, it would make sense to focus on how to exploit positive feelings.

True, the purpose of feelings is to orchestrate behaviour to maximise evolutionary aims; but from the point of view of the individual, whatever matters in life matters because of the impact it has on how we feel, not because it may facilitate procreation. We are in a position to dupe the genes. We can choose to make the most of the situation—to maximise our score of happiness—rather than to follow 'the wish of the genes'.

Having children can make you happy, but so can a lot of other things. I consider that to be a providential fact, because—for the sake of sustainability—our planet does not need an ever increasing population. To offer a chance of happiness to future generations, it may be better to focus on how to live a good life, rather than on how to produce many copies of your genes.

We have indeed a unique option. We are in a position to outsmart the process of evolution. Rather than to follow genetic objectives, we may seek happiness, and we can create a human society on this planet that allows happiness to be a sustainable feature.

According to generally accepted semantics, modern humans first appeared some 200,000 years ago (Balter 2011). The thoughts of our distant forbearers are lost; but we can follow ideas on happiness dating back to early written records. The Greek philosophers are particularly famous for their reflections.

Aristippus wrote about the notion of *hedonism* in the fourth century B.C. (Fig. 1.1). According to him, the goal of life is to seek pleasures. Positive and negative feelings distinguish what is respectively beneficial and harmful. As I shall argue, his main ideas still stand—at least if one adds the right content to the terms used. Other philosophers, including Epicurus from Greece as well as Carvaka from India, both living in the centuries prior to Christ, expressed similar notions.

Not surprisingly, some followers interpreted hedonism as a license to gluttony. Thus intellectuals, including the more famous philosopher Aristotle, eventually came to stress that virtue, wisdom and inner flourishing—not sensual pleasures—are the qualities that ought to be pursued. This school of thought is embedded in the concept of *eudaimonia*.

Apparently all the philosophers did agree on one core issue: What is 'good' for mankind ought to be the ultimate goal of society, and 'good' is a question of

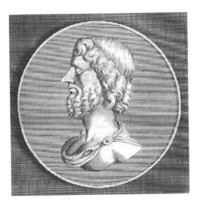

Fig. 1.1 The ancient Greek philosopher Aristippus (ca. 435–356 B.C.) from Cyrene (in present day Libya) established the Cyrenaic school of philosophy, an early form of hedonistic thinking. He was a disciple of Socrates. Although he is famous for his hedonistic ideas, he realised that one ought to show some restraint—as reflected in his motto: *I possess, I am not possessed.* (Illustration from Wikimedia Commons.)

processes going on in the brain—processes related to mood. They differed primarily on the question of what aspects of life are most suitable for making people feel good in the long run, and how to best help the individual in his or her pursuit, while at the same time care about what is 'good' for everybody else.

I shall argue in favour of using the term *happiness* for what is 'good'. It does imply a broader meaning of the word than what most people would think of as hedonic pleasures, yet it is restricted by brain processes that impact on our emotional life. Although the issues brought up by Aristotle have obvious implications for how to optimise happiness when measured over a lifetime, and how to make sure happiness is achievable for the entire population, they do not alter the main point: We should use our free will to depart from the course laid down by the principles of evolution, and instead focus on creating happiness on Earth.

The hedonia versus eudaimonia dichotomy—that is, sensual pleasures versus deeper values—is still a central topic when discussing what is important in life. I shall delve on the issue because it is important for answering the question of whether happiness is what we want.

Recent terms, such as *wellbeing*, *flourishing* and *flow*, are related to eudaimonia in that they are meant to depict a good life as something more than mere pleasures. The point stressed by those who prefer these alternative terms, seems to be that one ought to desire a successful life that includes aspects such as accomplishment and virtue, rather than simply covet whatever offers immediate satisfaction.

The dichotomy is an approximation. Different authors emphasise their own mix of constituents to be desired along these two broad approaches. In my mind, the discussion of what ought to be given priority in life concerns four issues:

1. A preference for immediate joy as opposed to a long-term strategy. For example, whether to gorge on food or focus on a healthy life for the sake of being happier when old.
2. Overt pleasures versus inner contentment. For example, to what extent one should go for external stimuli aimed at the senses or prefer internally generated cognitive activity as exemplified by finding a meaning of life and a sense of achievement. Note that both options promote positive feelings.
3. To what extent the individual should care primarily for himself—or work for the benefit of society.
4. Whether any feelings or emotional states are sufficient to be considered the ultimate goal of mankind.

The first three issues are primarily a question of strategies and means for creating positive feelings. I believe strategies aimed at maximising happiness as integrated over a lifetime should be preferred, and that the government should be concerned about the average happiness of the population, not the selfish indulgence of the individual.

Achievements and fulfilment of intellectual objectives are excellent ways of generating happiness. The same can be said for virtue and empathy. The latter statement seems obvious when considering the average happiness of all citizens, but being genial actually works to the benefit of the individual as well. In fact, it is reasonably well documented that positive social relations are a particularly important factor for happiness (Aked et al. 2008; Layard 2005).

The transition from tribal life to large scale society, starting some 10,000 years ago, had several ramifications.

One concerned the need for principles, or laws, guiding people toward socially acceptable behaviour. In a tribal setting, each person presumably depended on the others and consequently had strong, life-long ties with all the members of the group; implying that positive social relations were maintained. As the society expanded, people no longer knew those they interacted with; thus rather than relying on tribal feelings for maintaining cohesion, rules were required.

Another important change was the production of food beyond immediate consumption, as well as other items to be desired beyond actual needs—such as beer, jewellery and fancy gadgets.

These changes—the breakdown of tribal relations and the availability of superfluous products—would tend to cause conflicts and misbehaviour; in the sense of binge eating, drunkenness and fighting for the less accessible products. Secondary consequences would include a decrease in health and an increase in aggression. It seems likely that those responsible in society would try to counteract the trend by arguing in favour of restraint and moral norms. Thus to stress the values embedded in the concept of eudaimonia, as opposed to hedonia, makes sense—in the ancient Greece and perhaps even more so today. The availability of products catering to sensual pleasures has certainly expanded. Hedonism is, as might be expected, linked to problems such as drug addiction and obesity (Koob and Le 1997; Lowe and Butryn 2007).

In short, the cultural progression toward a preference for eudaimonic values can be explained by changes associated with the transition from tribal life to large scale society.

The guardians of moral values may, however, tend to overstate their message. Perhaps started by Aristotle, but certainly boosted in the Christian tradition, there is a tendency to advocate shame for those indulging in sensual pleasures and stoicism when confronted with pain. The children grow up learning to curb impulses directed at gratification, and to tolerate discomfort. Which makes some sense, but perhaps they should also learn to enjoy life.

Society ought to distinguish the pleasures that have negative consequences, and those that do not; as well as between unavoidable pains, as opposed to those that can be ameliorated. It is conceivable that the present categorisation is not based on state of the art knowledge—and, consequently, is not optimal. Our comprehension of the human mind has expanded considerably since the time of Aristotle or early Christianity. By disseminating relevant information, each person will be better equipped to make intelligent decisions.

The individual should be expected to follow his or her pursuit of happiness. What governments can do is to educate the population, so that the pursuit will be intelligent, and take actions that promote the happiness of all inhabitants. The latter implies to encourage empathy, to generate social capital and to setup rules that regulate conflicts.

Fortunately, we are a deeply social species; thus mistreating everyone else is unlikely to bring happiness. Unfortunately, people may be content working for the benefit of a particular sub-population—for example, the Arian race, or Catholics as opposed to Protestants—and thus find satisfaction in tyranny toward the out-group. An agency, such as the United Nations, that cares for the good of all is consequently required to maximise human flourishing.

Another issue is whether an impoverished person can be happy. Aristotle argued that a full and proper exercise of human capacities is required for wellbeing—so how about slaves, prisoners, retarded people, hooligans and couch potatoes?

According to the present definition, it is the lifetime emotional experiences that matter, not whether someone accomplishes anything or seems from the outside to have a fulfiling life. This position is supported by the Tibetan Buddhist tradition of looking at happiness as something that anyone can achieve by mental training (Lama and Cutler 2000; Ricard 2007). According to this tradition, it is possible to be happy and content even under the most miserable of conditions. Moreover, it has been pointed out that people with Down syndrome (Robinson 2000) and Angelman syndrome (Williams et al. 2006), both considerable mental handicaps, appear to be happier than the average person as long as they are cared for.

In other words, although aspects of life such as achieving something, or finding a meaning, can be excellent sources of contentment—they are not required for happiness. Both humans and other mammals can presumably be happy in the absence of these eudaimonic values.

The first three of the four issues in the above list can be included under the banner of happiness in the present meaning of the word. They do not contradict a definition of happiness as what society should aim for. The fourth issue, however, does not fall into this category. It claims that there is more to be desired than what directly or indirectly influences emotional life or feelings.

Belliotti, with his book *Happiness is overrated* (Belliotti 2004), is a prime exponent for the notion that happiness should not be our primary concern. His main objection, however, appears to be that having a meaningful and valuable life is more important than pleasures. This stance would be obvious if happiness was defined in terms of hedonia, but considering that the aspects of life Belliotti promotes are excellent means to obtain positive states of mind (if not always for the individual, so for other people), and consequently happiness in the present meaning of the word, then the question of what more should be desired seems less obvious.

A number of more subtle arguments have been raised favouring the notion that positive feelings are insufficient:

1. Creating more knowledge and a more advanced society is a goal in itself.
2. It matters whether our achievements are truly valuable for society, not just felt to be of value.
3. How a person is perceived after death is important.
4. A real, or authentic, life is to be preferred, even with its ups and downs, rather than unnatural pleasures such as those obtained by drugs, daydreaming or a life in cyberspace.

Again the first three objections can be squeezed into a wider definition of happiness—particularly when incorporating the potential for future people to have a good life. Concerning the stance that progress in knowledge and technical products is desirable, one may argue that industrial advances not necessarily improve the world, as exemplified by the weapon industry. Yet, the fourth concern is, in my mind, the more interesting.

The arguably most discussed version of this objection is based on Nozick's hypothetical machine that delivers any feelings or experiences one may desire without any negative side effects (Nozick 1974). Most people would not want to be hooked on to such a machine for life; they prefer the real thing even if it means misery and tedious tasks mixed with occasional moments of joy. In other words, even supreme happiness, if based on a 'virtual existence', is not desirable.

I would tend to agree—but would add that such a machine (or pill) is purely hypothetical and unlikely to ever exist. Based on current knowledge in neurobiology, we cannot devise a contrivance that delivers pure pleasure without any negative consequences (at least not within the foreseeable future). Happiness may therefore still be considered the ultimate goal within the scope of real life options.

Actually, the main problem may not be to have people consent to happiness (in the present sense) being the ultimate aim, but to coach them to pursue it intelligently. Even in the case of those who agree wholeheartedly, their actions may not reflect this stance. Their priorities are too often in the direction of short-term hedonic pleasures, rather than strategies aimed at maximising lifetime contentment—such as friendship, achievements and virtue. The rational response to this quandary is to distribute information as to what happiness is about; which is the main purpose of the present text.

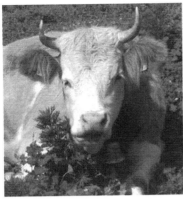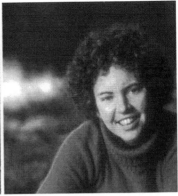

Fig. 1.2 All mammals presumably share a disposition for positive and negative feelings. In the absence of any cause for distress, the mood most likely reflects a higher level of activity in positive nerve circuits—a notion I refer to as a 'default state of contentment'. (Photo: B. Grinde)

Based on the discussion so far, happiness may be construed as the net sum of positive and negative feelings—preferably integrated over a lifetime. If the sum at any given moment is above zero, the person may be referred to as happy; and if the lifetime sum adds up to a positive value, he may be said to have lived a happy life.

I have already discussed some objections to this definition. One more issue is addressed below.

The suggested definition of happiness is necessarily a theoretical construct in that we do not have any objective way of quantifying positive and negative feelings. At least we do not have any figures that allow for proper arithmetic. Yet, it may be argued that the definition implies a rather low threshold for qualifying to be a happy person. Fredrickson and Losada (2005) have suggested that a greater than 3:1 ratio of positive to negative affect is required for favourable psychological functioning. On a similar note, I believe the propensity for life satisfaction is well above neutral for a mentally healthy person living in a proper environment, a notion I refer to as *default contentment* (Fig. 1.2) (Grinde 2002a, b). Consequently it may seem wrong to consider 'just above neutral' to represent happiness.

It is, however, rather difficult to set a particular value for the quantity of positive feelings required to be happy—not the least due to the problem of translating emotions into math. Moreover, my primary purpose is to present a model for factors that move people up or down the scale; not to try to define values or thresholds. I therefore prefer to leave open the question of how much positive emotional activity is required to be worthy of the label 'happy'.

I shall summarise the message so far.

My position is to define the word happiness in terms of positive feelings, and to construe that happiness is what the individual ought to strive for, and what society should work toward. It is useful to have a term for this purpose, and 'happiness' seems to be the best choice. It should be noted that the present definition implies a more comprehensive entity than the typical daily use of the word—in particular, happiness is taken to encompass both hedonic and eudaimonic elements.

Any preferred aim of mankind is an objective because it in some way, direct or indirect, at the moment or in the future, can stimulate positive feelings in someone's brain. The important issue is to deliberate on the suitability of various options in generating positive feelings. A bottle of wine, a solid portion of junk food, or a shot of heroin may seem more potent than the more eudaimonic alternatives; but when the effect is integrated over a lifetime, the virtuous choices are likely to do better.

Hedonism had its heyday, today it is frowned on. The sentiment of present Western culture seems to be that people should opt for intellectual endeavours, industrial achievements, creativity and, not the least, compassion and good deeds as their tickets to wellbeing. The old saying that making other people happy is the best way to personal happiness has a biological explanation—a point I shall return to later.

There are several reasons to endorse this stance, particularly when the concern is for the average happiness of the population; yet is should be noted that other, more traditional, pleasures may also augment the score of happiness.

1.2 Know Thyself

With the advance of empirical science, the old philosophers were relegated to history books, and the topic of happiness fell outside the scope of what was considered appropriate for serious inquiry. The subject was not forgotten, but advice on how to live was cared for primarily by the clergy.

Psychiatry and psychology were established in the nineteenth and twentieth century, but their primary purpose was to help people with mental problems. Only over the last couple of decades has a new line of research become popular—often referred to as *positive psychology*—which takes a more systematic look at the brighter sides of life. Psychologists eventually came to realise that the potential for impacting on people's mental condition is not restricted to those with particular problems; they can also help ordinary people in their pursuit for contentment. Furthermore, by caring for the mind of the average person, they may actually prevent psychiatric conditions.

Positive psychology is primarily concerned with empirical investigation of factors that correlate with wellbeing, for thereby to suggest practical advice. The point is to help individuals, families and communities flourish; that is, to make 'normal' life more fulfiling.

With this book, I wish to add another scientific perspective—that of biology—to the quest for understanding what happiness is about and how to promote it.

Traditionally, biology has been even further from engaging in human happiness than has psychology. True, Darwin himself wrote extensively on the evolution of human emotions and other mental faculties; but any concept in the line of 'positive' or 'desirable', any focus on the idea of success, would tend to imply *fitness*. Biological fitness is measured in terms of progeny—it is a question of survival and

Fig. 1.3 The ancient Oracle of Delphi was situated on the slopes of Mount Parnassus in Greece. The ruins, which date mostly to the fourth century B.C., are an UNESCO World Heritage Site. (Photo: B. Grinde)

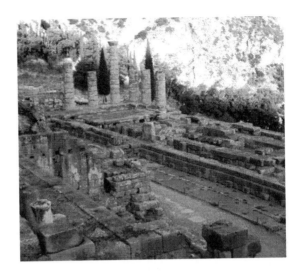

procreation—happiness enters the equation only indirectly. Yet, it is possible to use the evolutionary perspective to extract knowledge that has a bearing on the pursuit of happiness.

As a biologist, whose primary interest has been to understand how evolution has shaped the human brain, I have been engaged in this subject for more than 20 years. My first book on the topic (in Norwegian) appeared in 1996, and I have since coined the phrase *Darwinian happiness* for this way of looking at how life ought to be (Grinde 1996, 2002a, b).

Not only do I believe biology can offer meaningful additional information pertaining to the issue of wellbeing; but, as I shall try to demonstrate, the evolutionary approach offers a model that can unite the different schools of science and counselling engaged in this topic. A biological understanding of the human mind offers a framework into which information gained from other disciplines (such as the social sciences) can be added—and embedded in a deeper context. That is, I believe happiness does not make complete sense except in the light of evolution.

In my mind, the evolutionary perspective offers a framework for any question regarding human nature. In a way it means taking the Oracle of Delphi seriously— to follow their motto *Know thyself* (Fig. 1.3). And in order to know ourselves, we need to comprehend the process that shaped us.

The present text is not only concerned with explaining the evolutionary scenario that shaped the human mind, including our propensity for pleasure and pain; it also delves into the neurobiology of these feelings. Evolution and neurobiology represent two different biological approaches to understand the brain. The former offers a 'top-down' perspective. It tells us what the brain is for, but the working of this organ, i.e., how it performs its purpose, is left as undescribed territory. The latter is the 'bottom-up' approach. It explains the workings of the brain (at a cellular level), but needs the evolutionary perspective in order to make sense of the various functions the brain is supposed to care for. Eventually these two approaches may meet, and thereby enable science to present a more detailed picture of the human mind, but at the moment the 'white part of the map' that separates the two approaches is considerable.

The human brain is the most fantastic piece of engineering evolution has ever crafted. It is the one part of the Universe we really should strive to understand—as insight in no other topic can have a similar impact on our lives. For a scientist, however, it is a nightmare. It consists of some 100 billion nerve cells, an equal number of other cells that help the nerve cells, and trillions of connections between the nerve cells. The nerve cells may fire (send signals) from 0 to 50 times a second, and they form large networks that tend to fire rhythmically. During a single breath, 10^{15} signals move inside your head. The theoretical number of possible 'brain states' (in the form of which cells are active and where do the signals go) has been estimated to be $10^{1,000,000}$ (writing all the digits would require a book 4 times the size of this) (Hanson 2010). A figure that dwarfs the number of elementary particles in the universe, typically estimated to be less than 10^{100}.

Unfortunately, but not surprisingly, the brain is arguably the most difficult part of the Universe to get a grip on.

We may never be able to offer a complete account of what goes on in the head, but that does not mean we lack relevant information. The two approaches indicated above have made considerable progress; in combination they do make sense not only of what happiness is about, evolutionary and neurobiologically, but also of what constitutes a healthy mind as opposed to mental disorders. As will be discussed in Chap. 4, the more common mental problems represent, in a way, the lower part of a 'mood' scale going from misery to happiness.

One other aspect of well-being is worth looking into. Biology is primarily about describing a species—in the case of humans, the typical or average person. Individual differences are also of interest. Your chance of having a satisfactory life depends not only on the environment you live in, but also on your particular set of genes. The heritability of happiness will be dealt with in Sect. 3.5, along with what is presently known as to variants of genes that may have a particular impact.

For all practical purposes, the genes cannot be changed. Thus the factor we should approach to improve life is the environment. The biological model of happiness offers suggestions as to what elements of the environment, or way of life, we may want to focus on; as well as on how we may try to mould the mind. This is the topic of Chap. 5.

The present book is meant to supplement the understanding of well-being drawn up by the social sciences. I believe the biological perspective presents a more comprehensive framework, but research based on the social sciences is required to fill the framework with as much information as possible. The natural sciences are ill equipped to initiate the type of investigations associated with positive psychology, which has already amassed a considerable amount of relevant data. Moreover, the social sciences may actually function better when it comes to formulating advice that people can understand and utilise—possibly in conjunction with philosophy and techniques that first appeared in spiritual contexts, such as meditation. The strength of biology is in creating a theoretical scaffold.

To make the most of the collective wisdom of humanity, and thereby get the closest to knowing oneself, all lines of investigation ought to be examined.

1.3 The Evolutionary Perspective

As Richard Dawkins has pointed out, the genes are selfish units designed to maximise their own replication and evolution is the 'blind watchmaker', responsible for creating the most fascinating organisms for no particular purpose (Dawkins 1976, 1986). So, although the process of evolution is extremely good at forming ever more complex life forms, there is no obvious sign of intent. Yet, when describing the results of the process one sometimes uses expression such as 'designed by evolution' or 'the genes want you to'. These expressions are just shorthand for outlining the consequences of evolution, the genes themselves have no desires.

I am an evolutionary biologist, but my interest is centred on one particular organ belonging to one particular species: the human brain. This, unfortunately, is the most (if not the only) controversial piece of organic material for a biologist to engage himself in.

Social scientists sometimes claim that the evolutionary perspective bereaves humans of their free will, by giving the impression that our actions are a consequence of the genes and thus beyond personal control. This is certainly not the case. Our measure of free will is a quality bestowed on us by evolution—simply because it proved to be a success by making behaviour more adaptive. Moreover, the main motive for trying to understand how the brain has been shaped by the process of evolution is because that knowledge can help us. And the only reason it can help us is because we are shaped not only by our genes, but by the environment. As pointed out above, to improve quality of life it is the environment that matters, and the environment we need to focus on.

Those, like me, who address innate tendencies in humans, are sometimes accused of delivering 'just so' stories. It is suggested that with a sufficient amount of fantasy, a variety of evolutionary explanations can be used to explain any observed human behaviour.

In my mind it is not for science to prove anything, what science does is to create models of reality based on empirical experiments and systematic observations. These models will necessarily be simplifications, and they will necessarily be flavoured by the background of the individual scientist, whether it is biology or social science. The human brain is a considerably more complex entity than flowers or bacteria, thus the models created will be more uncertain. Although all sorts of 'just so' stories flourish in the media, the science-based models of the human brain are simply our best shot at describing this little piece of the Universe. True, the models are fraught with uncertainty, but they are what we got.

The accuracy of any portrayal of the human psyche depends both on the painter and the viewer. Thus a person trained in the social sciences may find models in this tradition more useful than biological models, because he or she is in a better position to see them correctly. That said, the evolutionary perspective has a lot to offer, thus one might hope that the social sciences will eventually include evolutionary biology in their curriculum.

I like the story of the blindfolded sages and the elephant. The sages were offered to feel different parts of an elephant and then asked to describe what an elephant is. Their answers depended, of course, on which part they got their hands on—for example, a tusk, a leg or a tail. In my mind, what evolutionary theory does is to remove the blindfold and let the sages see the entire animal. That should improve their chance of making an accurate description.

Evolution wants nothing, but as an evolutionary biologist I want to portray the human brain as accurately and objectively as possible. In this text, I am particularly interested in the features of the brain that influence our positive and negative feelings.

1.4 Some Words Require More Words

Over the past decades there has been a revival of attempts at describing the human mind, with all its emotional dispositions, in a biological perspective. The effort has been met with some criticism from the social sciences, but much of the disagreement seems to be due to differences in terminology: Both the choice of words and their conceived meaning reflect the different paradigms entertained by these two very scientific disciplines.

Humans were not created to be happy, and neither to be rational. The worldview people establish as young tend to stick. If you are politically conservative, you will read the news in a way that further confirms a certain outlook of the world; if you have a background in a particular scientific discipline, you will tend to evaluate information based on how it fits that paradigm (Pronin 2007). Unfortunately, few scientists have sufficient background in both social and natural sciences to be able to bridge the gap between the two.

I hope the reader will bear with my bias as (primarily) a biologist, and keep an open mind to the ideas I present. At the same time I would like this book to be comprehensible for people regardless of background. In an effort to make the text more accessible, and less likely to be misunderstood, I shall discuss the meaning of a few key words and phrases. I try to use concepts in a way that is compatible with both the social sciences and biology.

Happiness is a difficult word. Here it implies any sort of 'positive feelings' or 'desirable mental states'; and is, as such, what we ought to strive toward. The terms positive and desirable, however, cover a lot more than sweet sensations and outright joy.

How we experience feelings depends on what causes them—such as food, friends or sex—consequently happiness comes in many 'flavours'. The various pleasures may be divided as to their source or type, but it is also possible to devise broader categories in an attempt to explore the main constituents of happiness. Haybron (2008), for example, distinguishes between endorsement (emotional states such as joy in contrast to sadness), engagement (more in the line of enjoying the tasks one is up to) or what has been referred to as *flow* (Nakamura and Csikszentmihalyi 2009; Csikszentmihalyi 1990), and attunement (the inner tranquillity and contentment). Flow, and the related term *mindfulness* (Bishop et al. 2004), are connected with what I refer to as a default state of contentment (Grinde 2004). It is the good feeling that ought to be present when worries and other negative sentiments are avoided, and the mind is in a 'healthy state'. It is partly a question of being preoccupied with something considered a meaningful activity—an optimal experience stemming from a complete absorption in what one does.

Whatever divisions are made, it all seems to come down to activation of nerve circuits designed for the purpose of creating positive affect; a point to be outlined in more detail in Chap. 3.

Those who try to measure happiness—using questionnaires with items of the type: 'On a scale from 0 to 10, how well do you feel?'—tend to prefer terms such as *subjective wellbeing* (Lyubomirsky 2001) or *life satisfaction* (Diener et al. 2006). In principle, these words describe how satisfied people perceive themselves to be, based on both emotional reactions and cognitive judgement, with the added qualifications of whatever other facets of their minds that influence the answers given.

The term 'wellbeing' may, in principle, include both the impact of short-term pleasures and the deeper contentment that comes with a life well lived. In practice, however, it is often simply a term used for the results of the above mentioned questionnaires. One potential bias is that people tend to give more weight to the present feeling, rather than the 'net sum' of feelings over time, particularly in Western societies (Wirtz et al. 2009).

Another bias is to confuse success, for example, in economic terms, with actual satisfaction. A person who consider himself to have done well compared to his peers, may rate himself high on questions pertaining to well-being even in the presence of serious emotional problems.

Some scientists have developed instruments (in the form of questionnaires) that try to distinguish between positive feelings and a successful life. These instruments indicate that while the score for how good, in the meaning of successful, we perceive our lives to be does correlate with income; the more emotional aspect of well-being is hardly correlated at all (Diener et al. 2010; Kahneman and Deaton 2010). Unless these two qualities are separated, the answers to questions of how well we perceive ourselves to be are likely to reflect both.

Besides the issue of actual success in life, people may elevate their score of happiness because they like to be perceived (by themselves or others) as successful and/or happy; what is referred to as *socially desirable responding*. In some cultures, people value the reputation associated with economic success higher than in other cultures, the former will obviously tend to score higher on questionnaires that do not isolate this aspect from the general score of emotional wellbeing.

Apparently, the tendency to try to deceive others, such as the interviewer, is not a major problem (Piedmont et al. 2000). However, there appear to be a tendency in

Western cultures to report an exaggerated impression of one's personal mood (Headey and Wearing 1988; Hoorens 1995). On the other hand, the reliability of the tests for subjective wellbeing—measured as internal consistency—is generally good; and they do correlate well with other indicators of satisfaction and positive affect (Diener et al. 2009). In fact, even simple self-report measures correlate with intuitively relevant variables such as amount of smiling, physiological measures, health, longevity and how friends evaluate the happiness of the responder (Pavot 2008).

While individual answers may be biased, statistical differences between groups of people who share a similar cultural background probably reflect actual variations in wellbeing. Thus correlates with other parameters, such as social life, presence of nature and general health, may indicate which parameters are important for the happiness of the average person.

Overall, the results obtained by scientists probing subjective well-being should be interpreted with care, which implies it would be desirable to find more objective parameters. *Brain scans* offer an opportunity to indicate the level of activity in anatomical regions assumed to be involved in happiness. However, although scans have been used to gauge happiness (Davidson 2004; Slagter et al. 2011), perhaps even more care should be taken here. Our knowledge in neurobiology is not yet at the level where we can accurately delegate happiness to particular brain structures.

The term *quality of life* is typically used in connection with indexes that consider a number of factors of relevance for the happiness of a person or a population (Abdallah et al. 2009). The factors—typically including health, education, economy, social life, political freedom and spiritual values—are important because they generate conditions that help people flourish. Subjective well-being is often included in the indexes, but is the odd ball as it presumably reflects more directly the emotional status, rather than the relevant environmental factors.

Our brains are shaped by the process of evolution to care for a long list of functions, thus a useful descriptive approach is to divide it into *brain modules*— somewhat like a Swiss army knife (Fig. 1.4). Each module deals with a particular need that arouse during our evolutionary history, for example, directing movement of a finger, induce hunger to initiate food intake or bring about compassion as a way of building relations to fellow humans. Like the various tools of the knife, they can be engaged when required; but while the knife has a dozen or so options, the brain may be divided into perhaps thousands of modules. The actual number is primarily a question of to what extent one lumps related modules together or divides them into sub-modules. Furthermore, while the knife has distinct units separated in space, brain modules may engage dispersed neural circuitry and the same nerve cells may be involved in several modules.

The concept of modules does not imply an attempt to underrate the complexity of the brain, but simply provides a framework for organising present knowledge in neurobiology and psychology. Obviously any taxonomy of brain functions represents a simplification of reality.

Some of the modules evolved for the purpose of generating positive and negative feelings—what may be referred to as respectively *brain rewards* and *punishment*. The various parts of the brain involved in this task may be lumped together under

Fig. 1.4 The Swiss army knife, or modular, model of the brain. Evolution has added a long list of functions to the human brain. As with the knife, the various functions can be engaged when needed, but in contrast to the knife, the brain modules are not neatly arranged in distinct physical units. (Photo: B. Grinde)

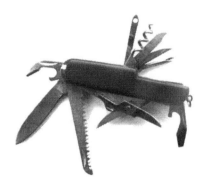

the term *mood modules*. *Pleasure* and *pain* reflect the activity of these modules as it is brought to our conscious awareness, and happiness can be described as the net output of the mood modules. Mood, in the present sense, covers both the delights and pains of sensual input and what may be referred to as temper or frame of mind. *Motivation* stands for the encouragement generated by the mood modules that is meant to instigate behaviour.

Note that, all parts of the brain involved in the generation of any form of positive or negative affect is lumped together in the mood modules. Although there is considerable evidence suggesting that the various mood sub-modules all converge on key neural circuitry, shared neurobiology is not a required feature for the present model of happiness. On the other hand, to what extent it is useful to single out a particular set of brain regions as being responsible for positive and negative affect in the brain, is primarily a semantic issue. We know some of the structures that appear to be involved, but our knowledge of brain architecture is not sufficient to outline all.

The conscious activity of the brain can be divided into a *cognitive* and an *affective* part. The cognitive part reflects in principle 'pure' thoughts, while the affective part is the feelings evoked. *Feelings* is here taken to include *sensations* and *emotions*. Sensations are reasonably direct consequences of stimuli arriving from either sense organs or homeostatic gauges—such as respectively pain and thirst. Emotions are more complex entities and typically involve interactions with other individuals. All sorts of feelings tend to hook up with the mood modules and consequently impact in the direction of either positive or negative mood—although the value is not always obvious, and often difficult to predict.

References

Abdallah, S., Thompson, S., Michaelson, J., Marks, N., & Steuer, N. (2009). *The happy planet index 2.0*. London: New Economic Foundation.

Aked, J., Marks, N., Cordon, C., & Thompson, S. (2008). *Five ways to well-being*. London: New Economic Foundation.

Balter, M. (2011). Was North Africa the launch pad for modern human migrations? *Science, 331,* 20–23.

Belliotti, R. (2004). *Happiness is overrated.* New York: Rowman & Littlefield.

Bishop, S. R., Lau, M., Shapiro, S., Carlson, L., Anderson, N. D., Carmody, J., et al. (2004). Mindfulness: A proposed operational definition. *Clinical Psychology-Science and Practice, 11,* 230–241.

Csikszentmihalyi, M. (1990). *Flow: The psychology of optimal experience.* New York: Harper and Row.

Davidson, R. J. (2004). Well-being and affective style: Neural substrates and biobehavioural correlates. *Philosophical Transactions of the Royal Society of London. Series B, Biological sciences, 359,* 1395–1411.

Dawkins, R. (1976). *The selfish gene.* Oxford: Oxford University Press.

Dawkins, R. (1986). *The blind watchmaker.* London: Norton & Company.

Diener, E., Lucas, R., Schimmack, U., & Helltwell, J. (2009). *Well-being for public policy.* Oxford: Oxford University Press.

Diener, E., Lucas, R. E., & Scollon, C. N. (2006). Beyond the hedonic treadmill: Revising the adaptation theory of well-being. *American Psychologist, 61,* 305–314.

Diener, E., Ng, W., Harter, J., & Arora, R. (2010). Wealth and happiness across the world: Material prosperity predicts life evaluation, whereas psychosocial prosperity predicts positive feeling. *Journal of Personality and Social Psychology, 99,* 52–61.

Fredrickson, B. L., & Losada, M. F. (2005). Positive affect and the complex dynamics of human flourishing. *American Psychologist, 60,* 678–686.

Grinde, B. (1996). Darwinian happiness: Biological advice on the quality of life. *Journal of Social and Evolutionary Systems, 19,* 31–40.

Grinde, B. (2002a). Happiness in the perspective of evolutionary psychology. *Journal of Happiness Studies, 3,* 331–354.

Grinde, B. (2002b). *Darwinian happiness—Evolution as a guide for living and understanding human behavior.* Princeton: The Darwin Press.

Grinde, B. (2004). Can the evolutionary perspective on well-being help us improve society? *World Futures, 60,* 317–329.

Hanson R (2010) The brain: So what? *The Wise Brain Bulletin.* 4.

Haybron, D. M. (2008). *The pursuit of unhappiness: The elusive psychology of well-being.* Oxford: Oxford University Press.

Headey, B., & Wearing, A. (1988). The sense of relative superiority—Central to well-being. *Social Indicators Research, 20,* 497–516.

Hoorens, V. (1995). Self-favoring biases, self-presentation, and the self-other asymmetry in social-comparison. *Journal of Personality, 63,* 793–817.

Kahneman, D., & Deaton, A. (2010). High income improves evaluation of life but not emotional well-being. *proceedings of the national academy of sciences, 107,* 16489–16493.

Koob, G. F., & Le, M. M. (1997). Drug abuse: Hedonic homeostatic dysregulation. *Science, 278,* 52–58.

Lama, D., & Cutler, H. C. (2000). *The art of happiness: A handbook for living.* Sydney: Hodder Headline.

Layard, R. (2005). *Happiness—lessons from a new science.* London: Penguin.

Lowe, M. R., & Butryn, M. L. (2007). Hedonic hunger: A new dimension of appetite? *Physiology and Behavior, 91,* 432–439.

Lyubomirsky, S. (2001). Why are some people happier than others? The role of cognitive and motivational processes in well-being. *American Psychologist, 56,* 239–249.

Nakamura, J., & Csikszentmihalyi, M. (2009). Flow theoy and research. In S. Lopex & C. Snyder (Eds.), *Oxford handbook of positive psychology* (pp. 195–206). Oxford: Oxford University Press.

Nozick, R. (1974). *Anarchy, state, and utopia.* New York: Basic Books.

Pavot, W. (2008). The assessment of subjective well-being: Successes and shortfalls. In M. Eid & R. Larsen (Eds.), *The science of subjective well-being* (pp. 124–140). New York: Guilford Press.

Piedmont, R. L., McCrae, R. R., Riemann, R., & Angleitner, A. (2000). On the invalidity of validity scales: Evidence from self-reports and observer ratings in volunteer samples. *Journal of Personality and Social Psychology, 78,* 582–593.

Pronin, E. (2007). Perception and misperception of bias in human judgment. *Trends in Cognitive Sciences, 11,* 37–43.

Ricard, M. (2007). *Happiness—A guide to developing life's most important skill.* Boston: Atlantic Books.

Robinson, R. (2000). Learning about happiness from persons with Down syndrome: Feeling the sense of joy and contentment. *American Journal of Mental Retardation, 105,* 372–376.

Slagter, H. A., Davidson, R. J., & Lutz, A. (2011). Mental training as a tool in the neuroscientific study of brain and cognitive plasticity. *Frontiers in Human Neuroscience, 5,* 17.

Williams, C. A., Beaudet, A. L., Clayton-Smith, J., Knoll, J. H., Kyllerman, M., Laan, L. A., et al. (2006). Angelman syndrome 2005: Updated consensus for diagnostic criteria. *American Journal of Medical Genetics, 140,* 413–418.

Wirtz, D., Chiu, C. Y., Diener, E., & Oishi, S. (2009). What constitutes a good life? Cultural differences in the role of positive and negative affect in subjective well-being. *Journal of Personality, 77,* 1167–1196.

Chapter 2
Evolution of Nervous Systems

Abstract This chapter starts by discussing the question of what type of organisms can be happy, concluding that it rests with the capacity to experience feelings, which also implies a capacity for consciousness. Within vertebrates, this feature is presumably limited to amniotes (i.e. reptiles, birds and mammals). Feelings evolve because they allow for a more flexible and adaptive behaviour. They have two primary values—positive and negative—aimed at respectively, instigation and avoidance. Happiness is a question of positive feelings. The brain employs the principle of a 'common currency'; i.e. the net sum in terms of positive and negative outcomes is calculated and used to motivate towards appropriate behaviour. Humans may have the capacity to be both the most happy and the most unhappy of any species. A main problem is that human feelings evolved in a Stone Age setting can easily cause problems in the case of a modern lifestyle.

Keywords Nervous systems · Capacity for happiness · Reflexes · Self-awareness · Emotions · Human evolution · Consciousness · Mood modules

2.1 Who can be Happy?

Creation of life appears to be easy. The first living cells probably evolved on Earth only a few hundred million years after the conditions were supportive for carbon-based life-forms. Based on our knowledge of the Universe and its constituents, it consequently seems likely that there is life elsewhere, and that it is founded on roughly the same chemistry; that is, it revolves around the atoms of carbon, oxygen, nitrogen and hydrogen. Unfortunately, due to the distances in the cosmos, we shall most likely never know.

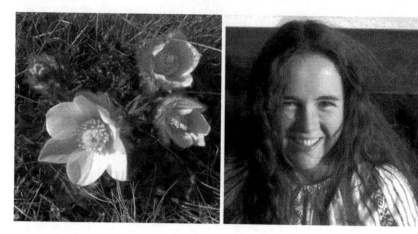

Fig. 2.1 What types of organisms can be happy? The answer to this question suggests what happiness is about. Here exemplified with a flower and a human. (Photo: B. Grinde)

Intelligent life, however, is something else. It took evolution close to 4 billion years to come up with an organism with the capacity to understand what life and the Universe are about; and of all the millions of species the process has devised, only one of them has this faculty. In other words, conscious intelligence requires a lot more to evolve compared to simple bacterial life-forms. [I have discussed this topic in more depth in a previous book (Grinde 2011)].

In the process of getting there, evolution gradually added a long list of features. The lineage started with unicellular life and moved on to simple multicellular organisms, through invertebrates, early vertebrates, mammals, apes and finally, humans. Besides cognitive aptitude, another of the features added is our capacity for feelings, including positive and negative affect. We tend to take our capabilities for granted, but a conscious awareness of feelings, the experience of pleasure and pain, is not at all that obvious.

If you ask people whether a flower can be happy, some will claim the answer to be 'yes'. They value their flowers, and offer them the best in conditions and treatment in order to make the plants happy. The effort may help the gardens flourish, which will make the gardener happy; but the plants are unable to appreciate the effort. In order to sense anything at all, a nervous system is required; a feature only offered animals (Fig. 2.1).

The 4-billion-year-long story of life includes only a handful of really novel and great feats of evolutionary engineering. One of them was the creation of multi-cellular life where different types of cells collaborate in the tasks required for survival and procreation. This process started at least a billion years ago. However, the more advanced results—in forms of size (being macroscopic rather than visible only in the microscope), variety of cell types and variety of life strategies—did not appear until 600 million years ago. The radiation of life-forms that occurred then was another momentous feat, and included the development of early nervous systems. There are still many animals around that have retained much of the features seen in this early fauna, such as nematodes (roundworms) and corals. These animals have nerve circuitry, so do they have the capacity for happiness?

Again the answer is most likely 'no'. Having a nervous system is a necessary, but not sufficient requirement. In order to answer the question of which organisms can be happy, it is important to understand the function of the nervous system and how evolution moulded it in the lineage leading to humans.

2.2 From Reflexes to Feelings

As multicellular animals grew larger and more complex, they required a system capable of organising and coordinating the activity of the various parts of the body. Nerve cells evolved for this purpose. They offer a fast and efficient way of signalling, with more specificity as to targeting the signals to specific parts compared to the alternative: simply passing around chemical substances.

The reason why plants never obtained anything similar to a nervous system is presumably because they (or at least the more complex versions) are sedentary. They do not need to move around to find food, as their source of energy—sunlight—is available all over the surface of the Earth. If anything, they would need to grow tall in order to be first in line for the incoming rays. Animals, however, are required to seek out their food, and consume a more or less limited resource in competition with others—in short, their survival requires what we refer to as behaviour.

Some animals, such as corals and sea anemones, are actually sedentary, but they either have tentacles that are used to catch prey, or they simply move the food (by moving the water) towards their digestive system. In other words, these animals too need the capacity of behaviour; which may be defined as movements required for survival and procreation. Plants in general do not. The nerve system, and the concomitant use of muscles, was the evolutionary response to this requirement.

In complex animals like vertebrates, the nervous system infiltrates all parts of the body. It connects with sense organs, to extract information from the environment, and effector organs (muscles), to orchestrate behaviour. The sense organs offer the organism information that is used to decide on an action, and the muscles set the action in motion. Between these two lies a processing capacity, which in advanced animals is referred to as a brain. The simpler, invertebrate animals have small masses of nerve cells referred to as ganglia, which takes care of their, more basic, requirements for processing (Fig. 2.2).

The design has been an obvious success, as it is found in all but very small and/ or primitive animals. The combination of senses, nerves and muscles allows the organisms to respond to the various challenges of living in an efficient way.

A nerve system does not imply a capacity for happiness. In order to understand the evolution of this capacity, one first needs to take a closer look at the challenges the nerves are meant to cope with.

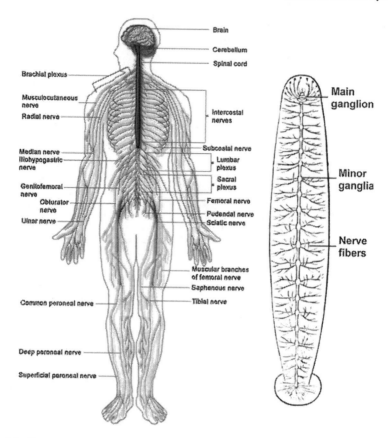

Fig. 2.2 Nervous system of a human and a leech (a segmented worm)—not to scale. The size and complexity of the central processing unit (respectively brain and main ganglion) reflect the requirement for flexibility and adaptability of behaviour. (Modified from Wikimedia Commons, attributed to respectively Persian Poet Gal and public domain)

Biologically speaking, what matters in life are survival and procreation. In order to succeed, the organism is required to go for opportunities, for example in the form of food or a mate; and to avoid dangers, such as predators or toxic substances. Another way of putting it is to say that life is about maintaining homeostasis—e.g. to find food in order to retain energy balance, to avoid harm to befall any part of the body and to retain a proper temperature—while at the same time try to obtain a chance to procreate.

The challenges facing an animal in this pursuit can, as a rule of thumb, be divided into two types: It is a question of either moving *towards* something or *avoiding* something. This dichotomy of purpose has followed nervous systems throughout evolution. The brain is there to help direct you towards opportunities suitable for promoting your genes, and to make sure you avoid anything bad.

In the early nervous systems the task was cared for by *reflexes*. If sensory cells reported the availability of nutritious substances, the message would be relayed to the appropriate muscle cells without further deliberation. The outcome would be that the organism moved towards the food source by following a chemical gradient. Some processing would be required by the nerve ganglia in order to recruit the right set of muscle fibres, but it is a fairly straightforward task. This sort of processing can be studied in, for example, present day worms, of which the nematode *Caenorhabditis elegans* is the prime toy for biologists seeking to dissect the system to its fine details.

Although simple animals like nematodes and leeches have the same basic requirements for life as does humans, evolution has elaborated considerably on how to solve the various tasks. Reflexes are fine as long as the exact same response is appropriate each time. Let us, for example, consider the task of feeding. If survival is cared for by filtering water pushed through a digestive system, then no advanced behaviour is required. On the other hand, when a leopard spots an antelope that may hide, or launch a counterattack, then the question of how to get that piece of nutrient into the mouth is far more challenging. To overcome such obstacles evolution created brains that allowed for more advanced computation, including the process of learning.

Learning means that the organism will base its response to the next opportunity on the outcome of former strategies in similar situations. If one particular way of dealing with a certain type of prey was almost successful last time, then the carnivore may elaborate slightly on the attack. Over time, learning offers a more versatile response to the challenges of life compared to reflexes.

In fish (and many invertebrates) some of the tasks cared for by the brain can be moderated by learning. As evolution moved on to amphibians, reptiles and mammals, the organisms came to rely even more on this capacity. Although we still find pure reflexes in the human repertoire of behaviour, for example how the pupils accommodate to changes in light intensity, in the case of more complicated situations we usually bring the task to conscious awareness and allow our advanced, computational brain to decide on the most favourable action. The decision will be based on both innate guidance and previous experience. In other words, evolution gradually added more power to the brain in order to come up with ever more advanced and adaptive deliberations.

Learning does not require feelings. Feelings were the next step in the evolution of more advanced decision making: *They were added as a means to evaluate various options.* If the opportunity is a simple 'grab the food while you can' setting, then the computation is easy; but in most situations there will be a long list of factors that point in different directions as to what actions ought to be taken. The better the brain is at weighing these alternatives, the more likely the individual is to end up with the best choice.

The weighing of alternatives requires a sort of 'currency' in the brain—a value associated with the various relevant factors that can be added and subtracted in the computation meant to end up with a decision. Positive and negative feelings were the evolutionary response. They serve as 'legal tender' for the (survival) value of various options–that is, potential pains and pleasures can be weighed against each other in order to derive at a best score (Cabanac 1992). The strategy may be referred to as pleasure maximisation, and in a natural environment the result will tend to be the best choice as to survival of the genes.

In the example of the leopard, the prospect of getting a kick from the antelope, or of not catching it, brings forth negative feelings; while the prospect of eating the meat brings positive feelings. The issue of whether to go for it or not, should be based on the sum of these feelings. The value given to each factor depends on previous experience (having felt the hooves of an antelope), as well as innate guidance (the degree of hunger).

Another example: When a human sights a snake there is an innate tendency to respond with fear (a negative feeling). However, previous experience, perhaps telling the individual that this particular snake is not dangerous, can neutralise the fear and instead let the positive feelings associated with curiosity decide on an action.

Before moving on with the question of who can be happy, I shall offer a brief discussion of consciousness.

Although learning does not require feelings, feelings allows for a more versatile way of learning. They permit the organism to take more factors into account, by giving the brain the equivalent of an algorithm to deal with the factors in a meaningful way—i.e. to add up their value. But for feelings to make any sense, they need to be felt.

This latter point may explain why consciousness evolved. Feeling a pain, as opposed to simply reacting to the noxious stimuli by avoidance, requires some sort of awareness—a sense of a 'self'. It is hard to conceive how feelings can function as legal tender without an awareness component. In other words, I suggest that consciousness evolved to give the animal the capacity to evaluate feelings. As the prospect of happiness depends on the ability to experience feelings, it requires a certain level of consciousness.

The early forms of consciousness probably did not imply what may be referred to as true *self-awareness*. Self-awareness, or self-recognition, is typically tested by the 'mirror test' (Kitchen et al. 1996; Reiss and Marino 2001). Here, an animal has to demonstrate that it recognises who its reflection in the mirror is. Apes, as well as some cetaceans, generally pass, while birds are more likely to seek the mirror for company, and dogs may bark at their reflections. Although these latter species flunk the test, they may still be endowed with some form of consciousness.

The sensory system designed to instigate approach or avoidance was installed long before evolution started to elaborate on how the response should be decided on. The capacity to experience good and bad feelings is simply the most advanced tool for decision making that evolution has come up with. Rather than a simple processing to redirect sensory information to the right muscles, the signals are diverted to brain centres evolved for the purpose of producing affect: A positive experience should spur an appropriate action, while a negative experience should produce avoidance.

The original feelings were probably based on direct input from sensory organs (both external, such as touch, and internal such as thirst). As I shall return to in the next chapter, evolution co-opted the system in order to generate more advanced, or diversified, forms of feelings, which include what we refer to as emotions.

Reflexes, or fixed action patterns, cause an immediate response, while feelings generate a motivation to act. The word motivation here refers to the 'conclusion' derived at when assessing the feelings.

In cases where a fast response is required, that is still possible. When you put your finger on a hot stove, the withdrawal works like a reflex; that is, you pull your finger back without any contemplation. You still feel the pain, however, because the pain is there to teach you to avoid touching the stove on future occasions. The example illustrates that an important rational for feelings is to learn how to best cope with future situations—to give the brain information that can be used to add the appropriate value to various behavioural choices.

Theoretically, a purely cognitive assessment of options (without feelings) would be possible, but evolution did not end up with that option for good reasons: Cognition was not sufficiently advanced in our early mammalian ancestors to make this a viable strategy. Moving from fixed action patterns, to learned behaviour, and on to motivation based on feelings is a more likely evolutionary track. It is more in line with how evolution is known to work: The genes devise indirect measures to cause their wrapping (the individual) to promote their propagation.

Early vertebrate brains presumably did not include true consciousness, thus the deliberations were originally of a 'semi-conscious' manner. Full consciousness (including self-awareness) evolved gradually as a further improvement of the process, but even in humans much of the computation giving rise to the feelings aimed at directing behaviour takes place in the subconscious parts of the brain. The transfer of power to awareness is only partial (Cabanac and Bonniot-Cabanac 2007; Pessiglione et al. 2008).

We feel pain in situations where it is possible to launch a response—such as pulling the finger away from a flame. In general, we do not sense the advancement of a solid tumour before it happens to push on nerve cells installed for other purposes. The obvious reason is that sensing a tumour would make no difference—cancer is not something we can make stop or learn to avoid (not counting the advances of modern medicine). Feelings evolved to impact on behaviour in situations where it makes biological sense.

The original dichotomy of either approach or avoidance has remained, and causes the feelings to have two basal qualities, good or bad. They do, however, come in a variety of flavours. Although they all have a mood value, they serve diverse functions. For example, it will do you no good to eat if your stomach has already been filled up and what the body requires is water.

Feelings are there to fine-tune behaviour according to what is most appropriate, or most important, under the circumstances. Evolution has consequently devised many ways to activate the reward and punishment buttons, and in each case the activation can be feeble or strong. Most likely there is a preset tendency to give priority to certain types of objectives. Thus, avoiding a minor injury is probably

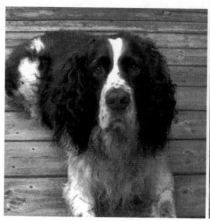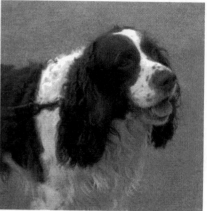

Fig. 2.3 Other mammals presumably have feelings related to those we have. The point is supported by the observation that animals share emotional display features with humans to the extent that we can recognise their mood. Here, the same dog as somewhat sad (*left*) and happy (*right*). (Photo: B. Grinde)

less important than laying down a prey. And if the opportunity knocking is a chance of procreation, most other activities should be dropped.

Based on the above discussion, we may be able to formulate an answer to the question of who can be happy.

Various lines of research suggest that the capacity to have some sort of conscious awareness of pleasure and pain, and thus a propensity for happiness, evolved between the amphibian and reptilian stages of vertebrate evolution (Cabanac 1999; Edelman and Seth 2009; Cabanac et al. 2009). A reptile seeks pleasurable stimuli, such as sunbathing. Moreover, it is possible to measure a physiological response in the sunbathing reptile, and the response is akin to what we can measure in humans when they are engaged in positive experiences. Fish and amphibians do not show the same response; their behaviour appear to be more instinctive and less influenced by an actual awareness of sensations (Braithwaite and Boulcott 2007). Birds, on the other hand, presumably can be happy as they evolved from the reptilian lineage.

At the very least we share the capacity for happiness with other mammals. The conserved nature of the corresponding mental states can be deduced from the observation that different mammals display similar affective expressions related to both liking and disliking (Hallcrest 1992; Steiner et al. 2001). We recognise the mood of these animals by their face and body language (Fig. 2.3).

Emotions are primarily a phenomenon associated with social life. They are displayed for the purpose of informing other individuals, otherwise the visual (or auditory) expression would not have evolved. In other words, emotions are presented to the extent that the display serves a purpose—for example in the form of chasing away intruders or obtaining support from comrades. The observation, that we can read the emotions of other mammals, suggests that the underlying neurobiology evolved early in the mammalian lineage. Most emotions can trigger the reward and punishment buttons in the brain, indicating that all mammals have the capacity to experience the positive and negative effects.

In fact, the happiness of chimpanzees has been assessed by human observers. The resulting score correlated with factors that would be expected to be important for happiness, such as place in hierarchy and stress level (Weiss et al. 2002). Similar results have been obtained with orangutans (Weiss et al. 2006).

It should be mentioned that opinions differ as to whether fish (and other non-mammalian vertebrates) have feelings (Braithwaite and Boulcott 2007; Mosley 2011; Sneddon 2009). There is no doubt that these animals can respond to relevant stimuli in ways reminiscent to what we see in mammals, for example, in relation to pain and fear. The issue is to what extent this response is based on true feelings. We do not know how fish experience their lives, but even if we could have gauged their level of affect, the answer to the question of who can be happy would still rely on a semantic choice.

In order to illustrate the semantic nature of the question, one may ask whether various animals have a nose? In the case of a dog, some people will claim the answer to be 'yes', while others may insist that dogs have a snout and not a nose. Fish have an olfactory organ with a shared evolutionary history to the human nose, but most people would probably claim that they do not have a nose. The point being that all (or most) vertebrates have features homologous to both noses and feelings. The features have a shared evolutionary background, but have evolved in different directions since the time of species divergence. Whether animals have a nose, or a capacity for happiness, is consequently a question of how narrow (in relation to evolutionary divergence) these terms are defined.

In my vocabulary, all mammals (and more likely all amniotes, which includes reptiles and birds as well) can experience happiness, but not necessarily in the exact same way. Our closest relatives, the chimpanzees, have a nose, but it is different from that of a human—so, presumably, is their emotional set-up.

It might be possible to design an advanced computational brain without any feelings, and thus without an aptitude for happiness. Many invertebrates, for example insects, have a considerable capacity to learn, and they display complex behaviour. The dance form of communication used by bees is an extraordinary example, yet it seems to rely solely on innate instincts (Gould and Grant-Gould 1995). Presumably, there are no true feelings involved. Their learning is rather a question of changes in the nerve circuits controlling action patterns with the result of modifying future behaviour. The behaviour in question may require too much computation to be referred to as reflexes, but is still covered by the term 'instinctive'. Instincts can be acted out without conscious considerations, and without the use of motivational instigation.

Actually, even advanced forms of behaviour do not necessarily require learning. The birds' capacity to fly, for example, is apparently not something the bird learns, but is rather a matter of maturation. If one restrains the wings of some of the chicks in a litter from birth, they will still fly at the same time as their siblings once the necessary muscles, and their control, have developed.

Combining a capacity for learning with an awareness of feelings presumably offers the most flexible and versatile way for the nervous system to orchestrate behaviour. It is more costly (as to brain power) than reflexes and instinctive behaviour, thus we only expect to observe it in situations sufficiently complex to make it worthwhile.

Advanced, flexible behaviour has actually evolved outside the vertebrate lineage as well. The cephalopods (octopuses and squids) appear to be highly intelligent. They have a relatively large nervous system—for some species, similar in size to that of a dog—but organised in a very different way. Only a small part is located in a central brain, the rest is divided between several (large) ganglia. Their capacity to learn includes navigating a maze, using tools, learning from each other and solving complex problems (Thomas 2011). In other words, octopuses apparently make decisions based on previous experience in ways that are more versatile than the type of learning seen in most other invertebrates.

The sense organs, and the basal dichotomy of the nervous system that distinguishes between approach and aversion, presumably appeared before the split between our ancestors and those of octopuses some 500 million years ago. Have these animals also evolved feelings and concomitant consciousness? Do they distinguish between pleasure and pain? If so, they too should have the capacity for happiness. [See (Edelman and Seth 2009; Mather 2008) for recent discussions on the topic.]

We do not know, but we may speculate. In order to install advanced forms of behaviour, the concept of feelings seems to be a rational strategy. It enhances the adaptiveness of actions. It may be possible to erect a complex and versatile response without any feelings, but based on our present understanding on how evolution operates, I do not see any obvious alternatives. Computers certainly do not require either awareness or feelings, but their construct is very different from what one would expect evolution to come up with. Given that the basics of the nervous systems are similar in octopuses and mammals, a convergent evolution towards some form of conscious experience of affect seems plausible.

To sum up this section: A capacity to learn, in conjunction with feelings, offers the most advanced strategy for ensuring flexible and adaptive behaviour. For feelings to make sense, an awareness of their positive or negative quality is required. In fact, the need to evaluate feelings may have been the necessary rational for evolution to install consciousness.

The complexity of the computational task needed to consider options, is best cared for by a unifying entity in the brain. This entity, conscious awareness, should gather all relevant information and make decisions aimed at maximising positive feelings. Humans possess the relevant brain functions in the form of mood modules. Other mammals have functions sufficiently similar to warrant the use of a shared terminology.

2.3 Recent Human Evolution

Our closest relatives are the chimpanzee, the bonobo and two species of gorilla (Fig. 2.4). According to genetic evidence we split with the chimpanzees some 5–6 million years ago, and the gorillas not long before that (Carroll 2003). Evolutionarily speaking, 5 million years is a short period, particularly when considering that large mammals evolve slowly. Consequently, we have retained a genetic similarity to the great apes in the order of 98–99%, but there is still enough change in the DNA to explain unique human features.

Even we do not have total flexibility as to the control of behaviour. The heart muscles, for example, are left outside of conscious control, because a more reflexive type of management serves the purpose. No advanced calculations are required, solely a response to the varying need for oxygen. Moreover, rendering the heart to the whims of the ego might be dangerous, because if it stops, or beats too slowly, unconsciousness and death may follow.

There are at least three reasons why evolution has not created a species with complete, personal control over behaviour:

1. Versatility of behavioural choice is only advantageous in certain situations.
2. Originally, all brain functions were on auto control. It is difficult for the evolutionary process to move far away from this deeply embedded strategy.
3. Cognition could end up serving some particular concern of the individual rather than the interest of the genes contained within.

A more parsimonious scenario is that evolution expanded on early reflexive or instinctive behaviour associated with attraction and aversion by adding mood value, and gradually increased the cognitive capacity for the purpose of a more fine-tuned assessment of select types of behaviour. In short, the four-level hierarchy of operating procedures detailed below seems to reflect the evolutionary strategy. The availability of a particular procedure depends on where on the evolutionary three a species is. Humans possess all four alternatives, and the choice of procedure is decided on by the subconscious brain and depends on the situation:

1. Reflexive behaviour.
2. Subconscious, instinctive tendencies or action patterns, including a capacity for learning.
3. Feelings and superficial consciousness designed for instigation or avoidance.
4. Higher cognition called upon when needed in order to further evaluate options.

As an extension of the above line of reasoning, it may be theorised that with the advent of self-awareness and free will, a concurrent enhancement of the mood values would be called for. Mammals presumably have stronger feelings than reptiles, because evolution points in that direction. The values attached to various feelings, and used in calculating preferred behaviour, expanded with the degree of consciousness. A solid dose of free will should point in the direction of more

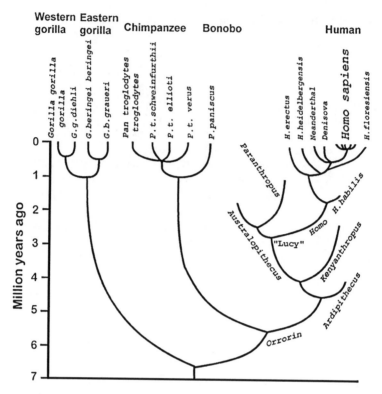

Fig. 2.4 Human family tree. While there are few fossil remains of gorillas and chimpanzees, the human lineage can be followed back to the time of divergence with the apes. Interestingly, 100,000 years ago there were probably six different species, or subspecies, of humans on this planet—today there is only one

potent motivational incentives, as the individual might otherwise use the free will to choose options that diverge from the interest of the genes. That is, higher cognitive functions imply a further gain in flexibility, but at the risk of ending up with behaviour that is less conducive to procreation. Stronger emotional incitements should keep the behaviour in line with the interest of the genes.

This conjecture implies that humans may have the capacity to be the most happy—and most unhappy—of any animal. The conjecture is supported by the observation that endorphins, key neurotransmitters in relation to reward and pain, are expressed at a higher level in human brains as compared to apes (Cruz-Gordillo et al. 2010).

There is one important caveat to the evolutionary strategy of relying on affective motivation: It requires that the instigations really point in the right directions. If the environment changes, this may not be the case. The recent availability of contraceptives is a 'modification of the environment' that exemplifies the point. We get ample rewards from our sexual activity, but readily dupe the genes by harvesting these rewards even when fertilisation is impossible. Similarly, the easy access to food designed for maximum stimulation of taste rewards will tend to cause overindulgence.

For the sake of happiness, however, duping the genes may be an excellent strategy—as long as the long-term prospects of health and well-being are not jeopardised.

Most experts agree that hominids evolved to live in a tribal setting. The tribe would comprise a number of adults of each sex, including several family groups, presumably totalling some 20–50 individuals. The members spent a great deal of time together and relied on each other for survival. Consequently, the tribe became a strong socially unit. In fact, humans have probably evolved some of the strongest innate tendencies to social affiliations of any mammal.

Interestingly, sociability has evolved independently on several occasions in the mammalian lineage. Although many species of monkeys are social, most apes, including the gorillas, do not form large groups; the exceptions being the chimpanzees (de Wall 2001). Both the regular chimpanzee and the bonobo are social, suggesting that the evolution of social life started in our lineage some 6 million years ago. Humans are unique in combining a highly organised social life with strong pair-bonding.

Research suggests that we are endowed with the capacity to retain relations with some 150–200 individuals (Dunbar 2009). In the Stone Age, the number presumably included one's own tribe plus members of neighbouring tribes. Neighbouring tribes would meet occasionally, as they depended on each other for exchange of mates, and probably traded information and tools as well. Only rarely would there be total strangers present, suggesting that in the absence of specific conflicts, an individual could trust the people with whom he interacted.

We are certainly more collaborative and empathic than the regular chimpanzee; and although the bonobo chimpanzee may be even more goodnatured and peaceful (de Wall and Lanting 1997), it is possible that humans have the deepest social ties.

The neurobiology and neurogenetics of mammalian social life has recently been reviewed (Robinson et al. 2008; Donaldson and Young 2008). Briefly, it is assumed that the underlying brain structures first evolved early in mammalian evolution for the purpose of bonding between mother and child (Panksepp 1998). The structures were later co-opted for pair-bonding (Lim and Young 2006). Additional bonding, such as between fathers and infants, and between adults of the same sex, most likely reflects an extension of the neurobiology used in these earlier forms of bonding. Thus, even though social life evolved independently in different lineages, the underlying brain modules appear to be related. In other words, once the neurobiology required for mother–child attachment was in place, expansion towards further social bonds could evolve relatively easily.

Both acts of aggression and acts of compassion can be highly useful for survival and procreation, consequently, one would expect them to elicit brain rewards. As I have discussed in more detail elsewhere (Grinde 2004, 2009), compassion—perhaps somewhat surprisingly—appears to be considerably more rewarding than acts of violence. This disparity may be related to the conjecture that the two types of behaviour were shaped at different periods of our evolutionary history. As discussed above, early on in vertebrate evolution, the behaviour repertoire was presumably instigated more by instinctive tendencies than by rewarding sensations. As consciousness (and the concomitant capacity for free will) expanded, incentives in the form of rewards became more important. Human social propensities most likely evolved much later than our aggressive instincts, offering a possible explanation for why hugging people seems to be more useful for the purpose of feeling good compared to hitting people.

In fact, the act of giving, as in charitable donations, can cause a stronger activation of the reward network than receiving the same sum of money (Moll et al. 2006). As would be expected, the rewards of giving, and otherwise acting with empathy, can improve personal well-being (Borgonovi 2008; Decety and Lamm 2006).

The main point is that social relations offer a rich source of brain rewards. The rewards include those we sense when falling in love, old love, being with friends and engaging in the fate of others with compassion. Relations are arguably our most potent source of positive feelings; a point underlined by research on well-being, which concludes that a social network offers the strongest, and most pervasive, correlate with happiness (Layard 2005; Aked et al. 2008). Besides being an excellent strategy for personal happiness, expanding on our propensity for compassion carries obvious benefits for society.

According to the present model, evolution intensified the role of mood modules in the lineage leading towards humans. Not only did the feelings become stronger, but the modules became engaged in an increasing variety of situations and behavioural encouragements.

This development may not be due solely to the regular forces of evolution, which primarily move in the direction of improved capacity for survival. The evolutionary process also operates by what is referred to as *sexual selection*. The peacock's tail is the most cited example; it is a considerable handicap in terms of survival, but evolved because the female birds came to prefer cocks with a large tail.

As humans began to understand the difference between joy and sorrow, they probably would start to prefer the company of those displaying positive feelings. We are able to read the moods of other people, and it is well known that happiness (and sadness) is 'contagious' (Wild et al. 2001). This translates to say that humans eventually may have considered mood when making partner choices—a notion that implies sexual selection. Thus, our present propensity for happiness may have evolved by a mechanism similar to that of the peacock's tail—perhaps without the associated burden as to survival. I have already pointed out that the strength of emotional instigations may correlate with the level of free will, an aptitude where humans top the list; sexual selection would mean that our capacity for happiness is even further elevated compared to other mammals.

The final major step in human history started with the invention of agriculture some 10,000 years ago (Fig. 2.5). Although early agriculture may not have improved the condition of life—that is, it apparently required more toil, and caused a

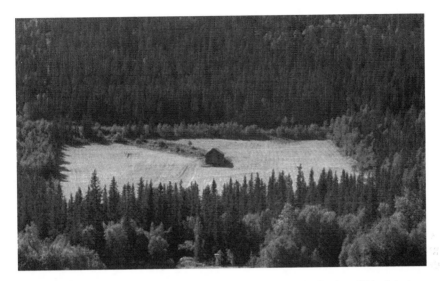

Fig. 2.5 Was the invention of our own gardens a step away from the Garden of Eden? And was the development of an industrialised society a step forward, or backward, in relation to quality of life? We have gained a lot, but we may also have lost something. (Photo: B. Grinde)

reduction in stature and life expectancy (Balter 1998; Teaford and Ungar 2000)—the invention eventually brought forth the probably most dramatic population increase ever witnessed on Earth. It also brought along scientific advances—not the least in the form of modern medicine—and, for a select part of the human population, a chance to live a life of comfort with ample food and resources.

Although the size of the human gene pool has expanded enormously, and with that the total genetic variation (in the form of rare mutations), 10,000 years is too short a time for selection to make much of a difference (Stearns et al. 2010). In other words, for most practical purposes we are still adapted to the life we lived prior to the invention of agriculture—rather than being adapted to an industrialised society. We live in what may be referred to as a 'human zoo' (Morris 1969).

In a traditional zoological garden, animals are removed from the environment they are adapted to; and unless the zookeeper takes the effort to compensate as much as possible to this predicament, the animals are likely to suffer both physically and emotionally (Moberg and Mench 2000). The question is therefore: Do industrialised societies cause human mental suffering by offering an environment different from what we are adapted to? I shall return to this question later.

The main points to remember from this chapter are:

1. The function of the nervous system is to orchestrate behaviour for the purpose of survival and procreation.
2. Feelings evolved because they allow for a more flexible and adaptive behaviour in that more factors can be taken into consideration when deciding on an action.

3. Feelings have two primary values—positive and negative—aimed at respectively instigation and avoidance. The brain employs the principle of a 'common currency'; i.e. the net sum in terms of positive and negative outcomes is calculated and used to motivate towards appropriate behaviour.
4. Consciousness was probably a consequence of the evolution of feelings, in that some sort of awareness is required to experience good and bad.
5. Happiness is a question of positive feelings. It is presumably available for all mammals, and to a lesser extent the other amniotes, i.e. reptiles and birds.
6. Humans may have the capacity to be both the most happy and the most unhappy of any species.
7. Social relations are a major factor in determining quality of life.
8. Human feelings, including the system of rewards and punishment, evolved in a Stone Age setting—in an industrialised society they are likely to cause problems.

References

Aked, J., Marks, N., Cordon, C., & Thompson, S. (2008). *Five ways to well-being*. London: New Economic Foundation.

Balter, M. (1998). Why settle down? The mystery of communities. *Science, 282*, 1442–1445.

Borgonovi, F. (2008). Doing well by doing good. The relationship between formal volunteering and self-reported health and happiness. *Social Science and Medicine, 66*, 2321–2334.

Braithwaite, V. A., & Boulcott, P. (2007). Pain perception, aversion and fear in fish. *Diseases of Aquatic Organisms, 75*, 131–138.

Cabanac, M. (1992). Pleasure: the common currency. *Journal of Theoretical Biology, 155*, 173–200.

Cabanac, M. (1999). Emotion and phylogeny. *Japanese Journal of Physiology, 49*, 1–10.

Cabanac, M., & Bonniot-Cabanac, M. C. (2007). Decision making: Rational or hedonic? *Behavioral and Brain Functions, 3*, 45.

Cabanac, M., Cabanac, A. J., & Parent, A. (2009). The emergence of consciousness in phylogeny. *Behavioural Brain Research, 198*, 267–272.

Carroll, S. B. (2003). Genetics and the making of Homo sapiens. *Nature, 422*, 849–857.

Cruz-Gordillo, P., Fedrigo, O., Wray, G. A., & Babbitt, C. C. (2010). Extensive changes in the expression of the opioid genes between humans and chimpanzees. *Brain, Behavior and Evolution, 76*, 154–162.

de Wall, F. (2001). *Tree of origin: What primate behaviour can tell us about human social evolution*. Cambridge: Harvard University Press.

de Wall, F., & Lanting, F. (1997). *Bonobo: The forgotten ape*. Los Angeles: University of California Press.

Decety, J., & Lamm, C. (2006). Human empathy through the lens of social neuroscience. *Scientific World Journal, 6*, 1146–1163.

Donaldson, Z. R., & Young, L. J. (2008). Oxytocin, vasopressin, and the neurogenetics of sociality. *Science, 322*, 900–904.

Dunbar, R. I. (2009). The social brain hypothesis and its implications for social evolution. *Annals of Human Biology, 36*, 562–572.

Edelman, D. B., & Seth, A. K. (2009). Animal consciousness: A synthetic approach. *Trends in Neurosciences, 32*, 476–484.

Gould, J. L., & Grant-Gould, C. (1995). *The honey bee*. New York: Scientific American Library.

Grinde, B. (2004). Can the evolutionary perspective on well-being help us improve society? *World Futures, 60*, 317–329.

Grinde, B. (2009). An evolutionary perspective on the importance of community relations for quality of life. *ScientificWorldJournal, 9*, 588–605.

Grinde, B. (2011). *God: A scientific update*. Princeton: The Darwin Press.

Hallcrest, J. (1992). *Facial expressions: Anatomy and analysis*. New York: ABBE Publications.

Kitchen, A., Denton, D., & Brent, L. (1996). Self-recognition and abstraction abilities in the common chimpanzee studied with distorting mirrors. *Proceedings of the National Academy of Sciences U S A, 93*, 7405–7408.

Layard, R. (2005). *Happiness: Lessons from a new science*. London: Penguin.

Lim, M. M., & Young, L. J. (2006). Neuropeptidergic regulation of affiliative behaviour and social bonding in animals. *Hormones and Behavior, 50*, 506–517.

Mather, J. A. (2008). Cephalopod consciousness: Behavioural evidence. *Consciousness and Cognition, 17*, 37–48.

Moberg, G., & Mench, J. (2000). *The biology of animal stress*. Oxfordshire: CABI.

Moll, J., Krueger, F., Zahn, R., Pardini, M., de Oliveira-Souza, R., & Grafman, J. (2006). Human fronto-mesolimbic networks guide decisions about charitable donation. *Proceedings of the National Academy of Sciences U S A, 103*, 15623–15628.

Morris, D. (1969). *The human zoo*. New York: Kodasha.

Mosley, C. (2011). Pain and nociception in reptiles. *Veterinary Clinics of North America Exotic Animal Practice, 14*, 45–60.

Panksepp, J. (1998). *Affective neuroscience*. New York: Oxford University Press.

Pessiglione, M., Petrovic, P., Daunizeau, J., Palminteri, S., Dolan, R. J., & Frith, C. D. (2008). Subliminal instrumental conditioning demonstrated in the human brain. *Neuron, 59*, 561–567.

Reiss, D., & Marino, L. (2001). Mirror self-recognition in the bottlenose dolphin: a case of cognitive convergence. *Proceedings of the National Academy of Sciences U S A, 98*, 5937–5942.

Robinson, G. E., Fernald, R. D., & Clayton, D. F. (2008). Genes and social behavior. *Science, 322*, 896–900.

Sneddon, L. U. (2009). Pain perception in fish: Indicators and endpoints. *ILAR Journal, 50*, 338–342.

Stearns, S. C., Byars, S. G., Govindaraju, D. R., & Ewbank, D. (2010). Measuring selection in contemporary human populations. *Nature Reviews Genetics, 11*, 611–622.

Steiner, J. E., Glaser, D., Hawilo, M. E., & Berridge, K. C. (2001). Comparative expression of hedonic impact: affective reactions to taste by human infants and other primates. *Neuroscience and Biobehavioral Reviews, 25*, 53–74.

Teaford, M. F., & Ungar, P. S. (2000). Diet and the evolution of the earliest human ancestors. *Proceedings of the National Academy of Sciences U S A, 97*, 13506–13511.

Thomas, V. (2011). A beautiful mind. *New Scientist, 11*, 35–39.

Weiss, A., King, J. E., & Enns, R. M. (2002). Subjective well-being is heritable and genetically correlated with dominance in chimpanzees (Pan troglodytes). *Journal of Personality and Social Psychology, 83*, 1141–1149.

Weiss, A., King, J. E., & Perkins, L. (2006). Personality and subjective well-being in orangutans (Pongo pygmaeus and Pongo abelii). *Journal of Personality and Social Psychology, 90*, 501–511.

Wild, B., Erb, M., & Bartels, M. (2001). Are emotions contagious? Evoked emotions while viewing emotionally expressive faces: Quality, quantity, time course and gender differences. *Psychiatry Research, 102*, 109–124.

Chapter 3
The Human Brain

Abstract All bodily components are vulnerable to malfunction, but the brain is particularly vulnerable. If the environment is different from what the genes are designed to live in, the risk of ailments increases. There are three core mood modules: seeking and liking (for rewards), and pain (for punishment); together they are responsible for generating affect. It is difficult to predict whether a situation, or a type of emotion, activates pleasure or pain. Fear and grief, for example, can activate either—depending primarily on cognitive input. The mood modules operate on a principle of 'common currency'. The concepts of anhedonia, pleasure-related analgesia and alliesthesia reflect this observation. The three core modules apparently cater to all sorts of positive and negative feelings, both hedonic and eudaemonic. If negative feelings are not activated, people tend to be above 'neutral' on a happiness scale—a notion referred to as a default state of contentment. Although individual genetic constitution is important for happiness, there is considerable room for improvement by optimising the environment.

Keywords Brain modules · Seeking · Wanting · Analgesia · Anhedonia · Alliesthesia · Emotions · Neurobiology · Neurotransmitter · Heritability · Setpoint of happiness

3.1 The Frailty of Brain Modules

The two concepts—modules and neural networks—are used for respectively an evolutionary and a neurobiological approach to understand the brain. In this chapter, both approaches will be dealt with.

The term 'brain module' refers to a part of the brain with a particular evolutionary function. Neural networks are the building blocks of brain modules, but the actual anatomical location and neurochemistry of the networks involved in any given function is, at the best, only vaguely known. Consequently, at the present level of neurobiological knowledge, an attempt to describe the brain in terms of its expected modules, and their role in caring for the individual, may be more informative than creating a map based on the suspected function of various anatomical regions.

Before I go on, it should be pointed out that evolution does not create optimal beings. There are lots of features in the human body that, if designed by a human engineer, would have caused that person to be fired. The spine is an awful technical piece of work, and our eyes are rather clumsily put together: The nerve cells are placed in front of the light receiving cell, causing a reduced sensitivity and a blind spot.

The reason why we are such a jury rigged piece of work is because of the way evolution works. There are at least six constraints that limit the quality of the result:

1. The starting point is an existing species and change can only be gradual.
2. The type of change is limited to what modifications (mutations) of the DNA can bring forth.
3. It is difficult for evolution to get rid of existing structures, thus the result tends to be like an old house that has been renovated and refurnished over generations of shifting styles—rather than a new house designed according to the latest technology.
4. Life on Earth is based on complex molecules containing the key atoms carbon, oxygen, hydrogen and nitrogen. The chemistry of these molecules sets limits to what is possible to achieve.
5. Evolution never needed to produce perfect species; it is sufficient that they stay alive and reproduce. The worst features disappear due to selection pressure, but the half good ones are often retained.
6. For a species to subsist, it is necessary to adapt to ever changing environments through the process of evolution. It is therefore important that the individuals do not live too long. The ageing process, with its deterioration of functions, is consequently part of our design.

The brain is no exception to these rules. The various modules are not perfect adaptations, but fraught with weaknesses of design. We can see this in how 'messy' the brain appears when we try to dissect the location and neurological basis of various functions; and we see it when things go wrong—in the form of mental disorders.

The human brain is also (arguably) the most complex piece of work in the Universe. Moreover, it is designed to be shaped, not only by the genes, but by the environment we live in. These factors, in combination with the weaknesses of design, imply that we are particularly vulnerable for mental problems. The situation is considerably aggravated when the environment differs from what the brain is evolutionarily adapted to—exemplified by a modern, industrialised society. Not surprisingly, it has been estimated that about half the population of Western countries suffers from a mental disorder at some point in life, whereas a third had a diagnosable condition during the last 12 months (Moffitt et al. 2010; Wittchen et al. 2011).

3.2 The Mood Modules

In humans, evolution has introduced an overarching brain entity, roughly speaking the cerebral cortex, which gives us a particularly advanced intellect, as well as the attributes referred to as consciousness, self-awareness and free will. A given brain module may involve both conscious and subconscious parts of the brain; and within the conscious brain, it may engage both cognitive and affective processes. Various modules presumably merge in the cortex, allowing the individual to decide on behaviour by computing input from several sources, and to have a unified experience of life.

Our intellect offers a chance to influence both conscious and subconscious affective neurobiology, and thus to some extent control how we feel. Thus, in theory we have the opportunity to manipulate the mind, and consequently our level of happiness, but in practise most people are swayed by environmental stimuli, as well as by processes initiated in the subconscious parts of the brain. In short, it is within the design of the brain to allow us to enhance positive feelings and diminish negative feelings; but having the desired impact requires special knowledge and skills.

The brain modules involved in generating mood or affect may be referred to as mood modules. They deliver rewards and punishment; that is, positive and negative feelings (Watson and Platt 2008). When brought to conscious awareness, we feel, respectively, pleasure and pain (note that the terms are here meant to include all types of sentiments, including items such as loneliness and sensing a meaning of life). It seems pertinent to define happiness as the sum of activity, or net output, of the mood modules—as it is sensed by the conscious part of the brain.

The term 'mood' should be understood in a somewhat broader sense than the typical daily use. It includes all sorts of good and bad feelings, and both short-term pleasures and pains, as well as the long-term aspects of temperament or emotions. Mood is here considered to be an aspect of the mind that moves up or down a scale from unpleasant to pleasant. Positive and negative feelings may be used somewhat synonymously with rewards and punishment. Words such as feelings and emotions typically focus on the particular functional role (e.g. hunger, love, grief or anger), and the concomitant 'flavour' of experience; while mood points to the actual positive or negative quality. According to the present understanding, there are independent neuronal networks caring for the particulars of each type of emotion and sensation, while they converge on partly shared structures responsible for their mood value (Leknes and Tracey 2008).

Positive affect is actually best understood as depending on two distinct primary modules, referred to as *seeking* (some scientists call it *wanting* or incentive salience) and *liking* (the reinforcing feelings associated with the actual consumption) (Panksepp 1998; Berridge 2003). Going back to the early nervous systems, seeking and liking presumably reflect two independent functions: The animals were instigated first to search for relevant items in the environment, e.g. food, and subsequently to devour the items. As these two functions were separated at an early stage in the evolution of the nervous system, they are expected to have distinct neurobiology, which indeed appears to be the case (Kringelbach and Berridge 2009).

The various mood submodules collaborate in directing behaviour, thus they are designed to influence each other. A minor pain should, for example, not ruin the chance for a major reward; thus the pain should be subdued in order to help the mind decide to go for the reward. Similarly, a small reward is not worth a life-threatening situation, and should consequently be ignored in order to secure avoidance behaviour. As reviewed by Leknes and Tracey (2008), various lines of research have demonstrated the above principles. Pleasure-related *analgesia* implies suppression of pain. Athletes, or hunters in former times, can be oblivious to pain in the heat of a chase. Similarly, various forms of pain (either physical or related to anxiety and depression) reduce or obliterate the capacity to experience gratification. The more chronic form of the latter condition is referred to as *anhedonia* (Gorwood 2008). In other words, to find the optimal motivational directives, the brain uses the 'common currency' principle when evaluating potential pains and pleasures.

Punishment and rewards may also be viewed as a question of encouraging the restoration of, or maintaining, homeostatic balance in the body; e.g. to consume food when blood sugar is low, and to avoid disruptive events such as falling off a cliff. The principle referred to as *alliesthesia* points to the expected correlate between the intensity of the activation of mood modules and the magnitude of homeostatic restoration (Cabanac 1979). Food rewards, for example, are more pleasurable when the individual is hungry, and a trivial fear can change to panic if the situation becomes life-threatening (Leknes and Tracey 2008).

The experience of pain may represent a deviation from homeostatic balance (Craig 2003), thus both the pain signal, and the subsequent pleasantness of its relief are expected to depend on the degree of the deviation (Leknes et al. 2011). Likewise, when a perceived threat becomes greater, pain unpleasantness increases, thereby enhancing the defensive response (Price et al. 1987).

It means that a main function of pain and pleasure is to encourage the constant optimisation of homeostatic balance. Although pleasure-seeking and pain-avoidance generally increase our chances for survival, it is easy to find situations in which these two motivations compete. One example is when a significant reward is accessible only at the cost of a distinct pain. The sign in gyms saying 'no pain, no gain' reflects this controversy. Again, the behaviour should reflect the net value when adding pain and gain, but in a modern environment, which is somewhat alien to our genetic constitution, the choice is often suboptimal for both genes and long-term happiness.

The conscious activity of the brain may be divided into a cognitive and an affective part. Cognition implies 'pure' thoughts and computations without any positive or negative value, while the affective part reflects the output of the mood modules. Obviously, cognition will tend to impact on affect, and vice versa.

Pain–pleasure quandaries are common in industrialised societies. [See (Leknes and Tracey 2008) for a further discussion]. Cultural values and moral systems are typically used to guide the individual as to which pleasures ought to be sought, and when pain should be tolerated. As the conscious experience of pleasure and pain is influenced by cognitive processes, cultural and individual ideas can have a considerable impact on how pleasant or unpleasant various stimuli or situations are perceived.

Most of the time, the activity of the mood modules seems to run at a steady-state level—we tend to experience the greater part of the day at a relatively constant mood.

When the steady state is disrupted, the change is likely to be initiated in the subconscious rather than the conscious brain. Although feelings are open for conscious input, once they reach awareness, it is not obvious that the mind is able to override the force of the subconscious. You can teach yourself to augment positive feelings, but you will never be completely free of negative affect.

The role of sensations, such as hunger, thirst, physical pain, sweetness and heat, are intuitively understood. Consequently, they are relatively easy to deal with, perhaps apart from the problem of overindulgence. The emotional units of the brain are more recent evolutionary additions, and offer a greater challenge both to understand and to handle. It follows that emotions are more difficult to exploit for the purpose of improving the score of happiness. I shall therefore delve a little deeper into the submodules involved with emotions.

As pointed out by several scientists, including Darwin, emotions are there for a purpose (Fredrickson 1998; Nesse 2004). The present use of the term suggests that their main purpose is to manage, or coordinate, our relationship with others.

Emotions presumably evolved from two different starting points.

Positive emotions arouse with the need for maternal care; that is, the attachment, or love, between mother and child. Maternal care is a defining feature of mammals. All birds, some reptiles and other vertebrates (as well as invertebrates) display various degrees of parental care, but the strength of bonding between infants and mothers took a giant leap forward with the evolution of early mammals some 200 million years ago. In invertebrates, the care is presumably instinctive rather than based on emotional instigation.

Negative emotions most likely served the purpose of dealing with competition within species; for example, in the form of anger or aggression between two individuals in the case of a conflict. Interspecies competition, such as between a carnivore and its prey, generally does not call for anger, but rather delight (due to the seeking module) in the case of the hunter, and fear in the one being chased.

A few key emotions—primarily fear, disgust and low mood—originated independent of social relations, but serve today both a role in relationships, as well as in their original, non-social context. Feelings (and emotions) associated with copulation are also of ancient origin, presumably they date back to a time when sex was cared for in brief encounters with no bonding between the male and female. In humans, however, the complexity of emotions related to sex is due to the personal connections between the individuals involved.

The human emotional repertoire includes a variety of items, but most of them are evolutionary offshoots of the primary emotions mentioned above, and the social nature of humans.

There have been several attempts at classifying emotions. One possibility is to consider a phylogeny; that is, to list them chronologically in the order of evolutionary appearance. Another option is to distinguish between primary emotions and composite emotions, where the latter is presumed to imply the activation of two or more primary emotional modules at the same time. It is also possible to distribute them in two-dimensional space; typically with the one axis being positive–negative value, and the other reflecting their strength or level of arousal.

As I shall return to later, one may also distinguish between emotions (and other feelings) based on how useful they are for the sake of improving the quality of life—either for the individual or for the members of a community. Empathy, for example, is viewed as a good emotion, while schadenfreude may be less desirable—when considering what is good for the community—even though both activate the reward module (Takahashi et al. 2009). Similarly, the sensation evoked by sweet food is less advantageous than sensations based on viewing a beautiful landscape, due to the different effects on health. The strength and duration of the activation of the reward or punishment modules is also a relevant parameter, love being more potent and lasting when it comes to enhancing positive feelings compared to, for example, anger.

In this chapter the main point is what sensations and emotions have in common: They are there to incite or influence behaviour, hence they have a positive or negative aspect. Sometimes the value is obvious, while in other cases it may be difficult to distinguish between good or bad. The good or bad part is cared for by activating the mood modules.

The human mind receives a vast variety of inputs. Some are initiated by the sense organs and reach consciousness via various processing centres in the brain; other inputs are internally initiated, for example, hunger and thirst as part of the homeostatic system. Most inputs—as well as the experiences, thoughts and sensations they generate—may connect with the mood modules, but only some have sufficient impact to be consciously regarded as pleasure or pain. In some cases the effect on mood can be significant, but is still not recognised as such, for example when a situation causes a person to worry without an awareness of the apprehension. In other words, the balance of activity in the mood modules may be swayed even without alerting the conscious brain. In fact, both external and internal signals can have an impact on emotions in the absence of conscious attention (Tamietto and de 2010).

In Fig. 3.1, I have listed important categories of feelings, with particular attention to those typically referred to as emotions. Many feelings can activate both the seeking and the liking reward modules; that is, it may be both a question of a desire and of a (subsequent) chance for consumption. The point is most obvious in the case of sensations, such as a desire for food evoked by sight or smell, followed by eating and savouring the taste.

Emotions presumably have a stronger cognitive basis compared to sensations. They require, or engage, conscious deliberations to a larger extent. That means that although all feelings, in theory, can be internally activated (such as when daydreaming), it may be easier to activate emotions than sensations in the absence of specific stimuli.

It should be noted that the categorisation of emotions is a very emotional subject—psychologists, and others, disagree as to what is the more appropriate list. I have offered my version, but realise that there will never be one correct categorisation as the brain is simply not organised in sufficiently discrete units.

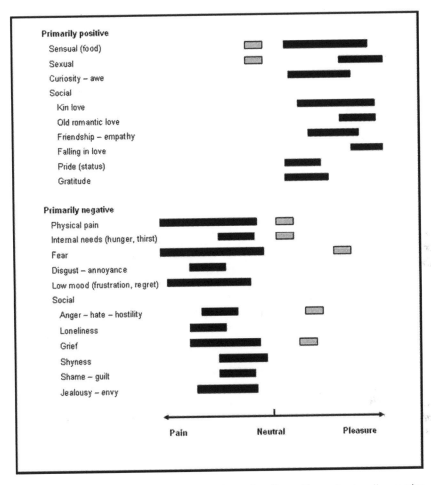

Fig. 3.1 To the left, a list of feelings divided into primarily positive and primarily negative. Examples are indicated in parenthesis, closely related feelings are added after a dash. On the right, their typical impact on reward and punishment modules. Grey indicates rare effects. The impact suggested is based on a subjective evaluation. It is not meant to be authoritative, but rather to illustrate a way of understanding the brain

I started out referring to anger as a negative feeling. I believe that in most cases anger ends up activating the punishment module, due to the frustration involved, but it can also activate rewards. Being angry can feel good. In fact, many feelings can activate either reward or punishment modules, thus their classification as positive or negative should be taken as an approximation. Fear is an illustrative example. In most situations the feeling is meant to be unpleasant (and consequently activates the punishment module), as fear is there to help you avoid harm. However, in certain situations it may be useful to face a threat; for example, in connection with hunting a dangerous animal. Consequently, evolution is open for a connection between fear and the reward module as well. Mountain climbers, for example, experience what is referred to as an adrenalin kick. The positive connection depends on the sense of being in control of the situation, if the climber should slip and fall, the punishment connection takes over.

Another example concerns grief. Normally this is a negative experience; it is evoked by events that are unfortunate for the genes, such as the loss of a partner or failure to complete a task. The brain reacts by marking the occurrence as something you should avoid. On the other hand, the reaction serves a purpose: The particular type of mental engagement may help you move on with your life; furthermore, sorrow is displayed for others to see, which suggests that it helps to communicate your feeling, presumably in order to elicit support.

The notion that grief may actually improve your fitness implies that, in the appropriate context, you are best served by engaging this emotion; and in order to instigate grief, a reward is called for. In fact, it has been shown by O'Connor et al. (2008) that although grief normally activates pain-related areas of the brain, it sometimes activates reward centres. The authors of this study suggest that the observation is related to the positive value of the attachment to the person the grief is focused on, but the observation may also reflect the notion that the brain stimulates grief as a coping response. Consequently, sorrow may feel both bad and good; which helps explain why people flock to movies that make them cry. When your own situation is not jeopardised, the reward part of grief may overwhelm the negative aspects.

Similarly, feelings meant to be primarily positive may sometimes turn 'sour'. For example, when we eat the fifth cupcake well knowing it is bad for health, and consequently punish ourselves for letting into the craving.

As indicated in the preceding discussion, and as suggested in Fig. 3.1, it is not obvious whether a particular situation will add or subtract to the level of happiness; i.e. whether it will activate the positive or negative mood modules. The context, the particulars, individual biases and certainly cognitive assessment, may move the experience up or down the scale from pleasant to unpleasant.

3.3 Neurobiology of Rewards and Punishment

This section is somewhat technical, but understanding the neurobiology is not required for reading the rest of the text. Moreover, most of the data referred to have a considerable degree of uncertainty. For example, the typical result from brain scans, i.e. a particular part of the brain displays increased activity in connection with a certain emotion, does not prove that this structure is responsible for the emotion in question. The scans do not yield high-resolution maps, and they typically reflect variations in cellular metabolism, and thus only indirectly neuronal firing.

The nervous system sends signals around the body by the dual mechanism of electrical transmission (by voltage changes across the cell membrane)—within the individual nerve cell—and chemical signalling (by neurotransmitters and their

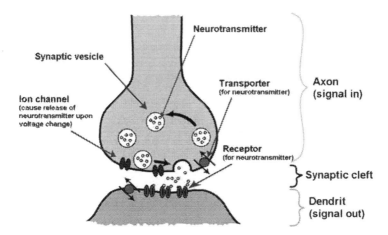

Fig. 3.2 The synapse between two nerve cells. The nerve signal travels through the axon by voltage changes. Upon reaching the synapse, it causes the release of neurotransmitters. These bind to receptors on the dendrite, and cause the signal to move on down the dendrite by voltage changes. (Adapted from Wikimedia Commons, author: Nrets)

receptors) to pass the signal across the synapse between two cells (Fig. 3.2). The nerve cells have long, thin extensions for electrical transmission. Those passing signals out from the cell body are referred to as axons, those triggered by neurotransmitters to send a signal towards the body of the next cell are called dendrites.

The specificity of nerve functioning can be cared for either by the wiring—that is, which cells connect—or by the use of particular neurochemistry in the synapses. There are a large number of different neurotransmitters, and an even greater variety of receptors and other molecules (mostly proteins) that can impact on whether the nerve signal is passed across a synapse.

The system allows for an experimenter (or a pleasure seeking human) to influence neurobiological activity by two different means: One alternative is to apply an electrical field to, more or less, specific areas of the brain. This can be achieved by inserting electrodes, but also non-invasively by, for example, transcranial magnetic stimulation.

The other alternative is to use chemicals that interfere with the activity of neurotransmitters. The substances in question are referred to as *psychoactive*, and include both narcotics and medicine used to treat mental disorders. As certain brain modules rely on particular neurotransmitter-receptor systems, chemical interference allows for a certain level of specificity; for example, benzodiazepines (such as Valium) act as agonists to the natural neurotransmitter GABA and are used in the treatment of anxiety. In order to have further control of the effect, the agent in question could be administered directly to the desired part of the brain—which is possible, but not practical except for laboratory studies of animals.

All mammalian brains include homologues of the brain structures understood to be involved in rewards and punishment (Panksepp 1998). Some of the main neurotransmitters involved in the mood modules—*dopamine, serotonin* and *opioids*—are used in even the most primitive neural systems such as that of the nematodes. Interestingly, they apparently serve the homologue functions of attraction and avoidance in these animals (Chase and Koelle 2007; Nieto-Fernandez et al. 2009). This observation further strengthens the idea that the human mood modules represent an evolutionary expansion of processes that have always been at the core of nervous systems.

The anatomical features of the human brain are traceable only to other vertebrate brains.

There has been considerable work aimed at defining the neuroanatomy of mood modules (Fig. 3.3). The more ancient, presumably subconscious, neural circuitry involved is situated in the subcortical part of the brain—particularly in the thalamus, hypothalamus, amygdala and hippocampus. The cognitive extension appears to involve circuitry in the orbitofrontal, lateral prefrontal, insular and anterior cingulate parts of the cortex. The subcortical nerve circuits are probably essential for initiating positive and negative feelings, while the cortex enables both the particulars of how they are perceived, and a capacity to modulate their impact. [See (Leknes and Tracey 2008) and references therein.]

As already pointed out, the two reward modules (seeking and liking) and the punishment module presumably evolved from simple neurological structures catering to approach and avoidance reflexes in primitive animals. Apparently all three modules have retained a partly shared neurobiology, both as to the anatomical features and the neurochemistry involved (Leknes and Tracey 2008; Kringelbach and Berridge 2009). The observation testifies not only to their common evolutionary origin, but also to the need for a close collaboration between rewards and punishment in order to derive at optimal behavioural motivation.

Although the three modules are partly co-located in the brain, it is possible to describe distinct features. For example, the opioid system serves a key role in liking, while dopaminergic nerve cells are important in the seeking module. In other words, dopamine motivates the individual while opioids are responsible for the rewards associated with consumption (Barbano and Cador 2007).

Pain and pleasure are entangled in the common purpose of organising behaviour. Decisions made by an individual are expected to be based on the premise that anything that is potentially more important for survival than pain should cause analgesia (pain reduction) (Fields 2007). This allows the animal, or person, to ignore the pain and attend to the more important opportunity. It is assumed that the analgesic effect is mediated by a pain modulator system located in the brainstem. The circuits here communicate with neurons in the prefrontal cortex, hypothalamus and amygdala in order to control afferent (inward) pain signals coming from the peripheral nervous system (Leknes and Tracey 2008). Endogenous opioids are involved in this analgesic function, and opioid drugs, including morphine, can hijack the system. The opioids are consequently involved in both the liking (consuming) part of the reward system, and in the pain module.

Evidence of pleasure-related analgesia has been reported in several studies involving either humans or animals. Analgesia is achieved, for example, by

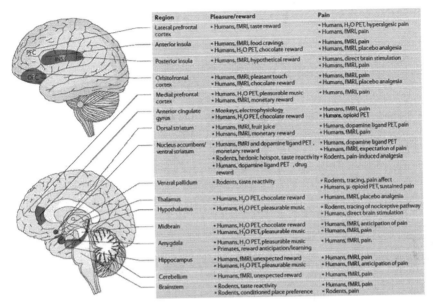

Region	Pleasure/reward	Pain
Lateral prefrontal cortex	• Humans, fMRI, taste reward	• Humans, H₂O PET, hyperalgesic pain • Humans, fMRI, pain
Anterior insula	• Humans, fMRI, food cravings • Humans, H₂O PET, chocolate reward	• Humans, fMRI, pain • Humans, fMRI, placebo analgesia
Posterior insula	• Humans, fMRI, hypothetical reward	• Humans, direct brain stimulation • Humans, fMRI, pain
Orbitofrontal cortex	• Humans, fMRI, pleasant touch • Humans, fMRI, chocolate reward	• Humans, fMRI, pain • Humans, fMRI, placebo analgesia
Medial prefrontal cortex	• Humans, H₂O PET, pleasurable music • Humans, fMRI, monetary reward	• Humans, fMRI, pain
Anterior cingulate gyrus	• Monkeys, electrophysiology • Humans, H₂O PET, chocolate reward	• Humans, fMRI, pain • Humans, opioid PET
Dorsal striatum	• Humans, fMRI, fruit juice • Humans, fMRI, monetary reward	• Humans, dopamine ligand PET, pain • Humans, fMRI, pain
Nucleus accumbens/ventral striatum	• Humans, fMRI and dopamine ligand PET, monetary reward • Rodents, hedonic hotspot, taste reactivity • Humans, dopamine ligand PET, drug reward	• Humans, dopamine ligand PET • Humans, fMRI, expectation of pain • Rodents, pain-induced analgesia
Ventral pallidum	• Rodents, taste reactivity	• Rodents, tracing, pain affect • Humans, μ-opioid PET, sustained pain
Thalamus	• Humans, H₂O PET, chocolate reward	• Humans, fMRI, placebo analgesia
Hypothalamus	• Humans, H₂O PET, pleasurable music	• Rodents, tracing of nociceptive pathway • Humans, direct brain stimulation
Midbrain	• Humans, H₂O PET, chocolate reward • Humans, H₂O PET, pleasurable music	• Humans, fMRI, anticipation of pain • Humans, fMRI, pain
Amygdala	• Humans, H₂O PET, pleasurable music • Primates, reward anticipation/learning	• Humans, fMRI, pain.
Hippocampus	• Humans, fMRI, unexpected reward • Humans, H₂O PET, pleasurable music	• Humans, fMRI, pain • Humans, fMRI, anticipation of pain
Cerebellum	• Humans, fMRI, unexpected reward	• Humans, fMRI, pain
Brainstem	• Rodents, taste reactivity • Rodents, conditioned place preference	• Humans, fMRI, pain • Rodents, pain

Fig. 3.3 Brain regions implicated in the generation of pleasure and pain. The evidence (including the experimental species, the methods, and the type of causal stimuli) is indicated to the *right*. A main point is that the same regions are involved in both pleasure and pain; and, although the evidence is primarily based on humans and rodents, the functions are presumably similarly located in other mammals. The *top drawing* is the left hemisphere of the brain as seen from the outside, while at the *bottom* the brain is sliced through the middle. fMRI: functional magnetic resonance imaging; PET: positron emission tomography. (Adapted with permission from Leknes and Tracey (2008), where further references can be found.)

pleasant odours (Villemure et al. 2003), music (Roy et al. 2008), good food (Reboucas et al. 2005), sexual behaviour (Forsberg et al. 1987) and possibly even the presence of greenery (Grinde and Patil 2009). Pain reduction due to the placebo effect is apparently also a consequence of the same neurological mechanism; in that the administration of placebo pills cause 'reward' expectation in the form of improvement of the condition (Petrovic et al. 2005).

A related phenomenon is the ability of pain to reduce pleasure. By inhibiting the activity of reward circuits, pain and other threatening events ensure that necessary action is taken to the effect of protection. It is, for example, difficult to enjoy anything if in a situation that causes intense fear; an effect also seen in the loss of appetite associated with pain (Stevenson et al. 2006). Morphine reduces pain, but the pain also reduces the rewarding effect of this medicine. The inhibition of rewards is probably due to activation of the κ-opioid system in the nucleus accumbens, and may explain why the medical use of morphine is less likely to cause addiction compared to a person experimenting with heroin (Narita et al. 2005).

The comorbidity of chronic pain and depression observed in humans (Berna et al. 2010; McWilliams et al. 2004) may be related to the inability of a person suffering from pain to enjoy everyday pleasures.

Although the opioid (liking) and dopamine (seeking) systems are closely related neuroanatomically, they interact in complex ways (Leknes and Tracey 2008). For example, phasic (intermittent) dopamine activity has been shown to increase opioid levels, whereas tonic (continuous) dopamine decreases opioid levels. Conversely, opioids up-regulate phasic dopamine in the striatum, but apparently down-regulate slower striatal dopamine signalling.

The interactions of the neurotransmitters involved, and the co-localisation of the various mood modules in the brain, support the idea of a 'common currency' for mood (Cabanac 1979). Regions that are particularly well situated to mediate interactions between pain and pleasure include the nucleus accumbens, the pallidum and the amygdala. These regions receive reward-related signals from dopamine neurons in the midbrain (either directly or by way of other brain regions), and are thought to signal errors in reward prediction (discrepancy between the expected and the received reward); as well as the actual hedonic value of a reward (Leknes and Tracey 2008).

Recently, data offering further information as to the neurobiology of the seeking module have been obtained (Stuber et al. 2011). While the basolateral part of the amygdala is important for processing both positive and negative affect, a pathway based on the neurotransmitter glutamic acid, going from this part of the amygdala and to the nucleus accumbens, promotes motivational responses (seeking behaviour). The effect is in conjunction with dopamine based signalling in the nucleus accumbens.

The most important point for this discussion is that the three mood modules appear to cater to all sorts of pleasures and pains (Fig. 3.4). In other words, the ups and downs associated with the emotional response to sociopsychological events rely on much the same neural circuitry that underlies the typical pain and pleasures caused by physical stimuli. For example, experiencing envy of another person's success activates pain-related circuitry, whereas experiencing delight at someone else's misfortune (what is referred to as schadenfreude), activates reward-related neural circuits (Takahashi et al. 2009; Lieberman and Eisenberger 2009). Similarly, feeling excluded or being treated unfairly activates pain-related neural regions (O'Connor et al. 2008; Eisenberger et al. 2003). On the other hand, positive social feelings, such as getting a good reputation, fairness and being cooperative, offers rewards similar to those one gets from desirable food (Tabibnia et al. 2008; Tabibnia and Lieberman 2007; Izuma et al. 2008, 2010). And the same reward-related brain regions are activated when having sex or enjoying music (Blood and Zatorre 2001).

Apparently, the ancient reward and punishment circuits of the brain have simply been co-opted for whatever novel needs that arouse in the evolutionary lineage leading toward humans. In other words, brain mechanisms involved in the instigation of fundamental behaviour, such as eating or sex, also cater to behaviour considered specific for humans, such as enjoying music or gossiping.

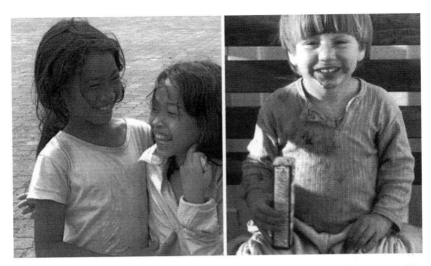

Fig. 3.4 Friendship apparently activates partly the same reward nerve circuitry of the brain as does eating chocolate. The mood modules have ancient origins, but have been co-opted more recently to care for the variety of functions required in human life. (Photo: B. Grinde)

The point is further underlined by the following observation. Although several parts of the brain are involved when sensing pleasure, only a few hotspots are known that will cause activation, in the form of enhanced pleasure, upon relevant stimulation (either electrodes or local injection of neurotransmitter modulators) (Smith and Berridge 2007; Pecina 2008; Kringelbach and Berridge 2010). These hotspots are found only in subcortical structures such as the nucleus accumbens and the ventral pallidum. They are neurobiologically connected, and presumably form a functional unit with strong links to the relevant cortical regions. The same hotspots, which may be in the order of 1 mm^3 large, appear to be involved in both liking and seeking, but while opioids and cannabinoids stimulate liking, dopamine amplifies seeking. As might be expected, lesions or dysregulation in these regions are associated with anhedonia (Miller et al. 2006; Schlaepfer et al. 2008).

The location of the hotspots supports a model where the mood "motor" is located in subcortical structures, whereas certain cortical regions acts like a "dashboard".

The cortex located, cognitive component of the system presumably expanded to accommodate novel applications, while the subcortical (motor) elements of the modules were retained. The subcortical elements may deliver a continuous tonus of positive and negative feelings, which moves up and down on the mood scale depending on the situation. The cortex adds the 'flavour' associated with the various experiences. A good meal, for example, produces a rather different impression compared to the joy of an aesthetic object; yet the 'affect part' of the pleasure may in both cases be cared for by the same reward circuitry.

Brain punishment, in the form of pain or negative affect, implies subjective distress and dissatisfaction. It is associated with a broad range of emotions—including fear, sadness, anger, guilt, jealousy and nausea—and consequently has a similar range of 'flavours'. Brain rewards, in the form of pleasure or positive affect, may include not only explicit happiness, but also feelings associated with being interested, energetic, confident, and optimistic.

The notion that various positive and negative affects reflect evolutionary developments based on a common platform is in line with our understanding of how evolution operates. In order to evolve novel features, evolution needs to start with a suitable structure that can be remodelled in small steps. A car manufacturer may decide to make a whole new type of car, for example, one based on electricity instead of combustion. Evolution cannot perform that sort of trick—it can only create novel versions by stepwise improvement of an existing structure. The case for the mood modules makes sense as it is possible to envision a continuous evolutionary production line, starting with the aversion/incitement modules of primitive nervous systems, and ending with the vastly more complex human mood modules.

The lack of pleasure is associated with negative mood and depression, while positive affect is considered the hallmark of well-being (Ashby et al. 1999). Both are consequences of activity of the mood modules, where certain key neurotransmitters and brain regions orchestrate the process of creating motivation and subsequent behaviour.

It is important to note that the cognitive impact on these modules can be considerable; both to the improvement and deterioration of mood. We can make tedious, or even painful, experiences agreeable; for example by associating them with something 'meaningful', or with the prospect of good times later in life. We may also ruminate on inconsequential negative thoughts to the extent that it obliterates any conceivable pleasure.

3.4 Hedonia and Eudaimonia

Based on the information presented in this chapter, it is possible to take a closer look at the two classical concepts related to happiness: hedonia and eudaemonia.

According to the present model, there are two main modules for pleasure—seeking and liking—but these two modules do not correspond to the dichotomy of hedonia and eudaemonia. One possibility is that the two reward modules only relate to hedonia, and that eudaemonia, or 'higher' forms of contentment, operates via unrelated structures in the brain. As will be discussed below, this assumption seems implausible.

Evolution is prudent, and generally operates by expanding on existing structures. Rather than devising two independent systems aimed at putting the mind in a positive state, one would expect that the original modules (seeking and liking) are expanded to take on novel functions. As pointed out above, the neurological template for reward appears to be involved in all sorts of pleasures, including those often cited to be of eudaemonic character such as love and compassion. There is no sign of an alternative neurobiology for contentment. A more parsimonious model is therefore that eudaemonia reflects activity that converges on the same neural networks as hedonic pleasures.

The observation that people suffering from anhedonia have reduced ability to experience all sorts of happiness or contentment (Kringelbach and Berridge 2009; Gorwood 2008), further supports the contention that hedonia and eudaemonia are based on the same neurobiology.

While the early nervous systems responded primarily to the basal requirements of life (e.g. dangers, food and mating), the complexity and repertoire of behavioural instigations have expanded enormously. One of the foremost items related to eudaemonia is to be engaged in 'meaningful' activities. It seems rational for evolution to attach positive feelings to utility, which implies that we are rewarded for doing something considered constructive. Thus 'meaning' is presumably a feature installed to avoid having our ancestors turn into 'cave potatoes', and consequently links up with the reward module. Originally, 'constructive' would imply 'good for the gene'; but today this gateway to brain rewards can be hijacked by all sorts of activities, from collecting stamps to playing chess.

Similar reasoning applies to other values typically incorporated in eudaemonia, such as spiritual associations, being virtuous and obeying social rules. Evolutionary speaking the ultimate objective should be survival and procreation, but all sorts of more proximate purposes may activate reward modules. In other words, the positive affect labelled as eudaemonia may simply reflect a subset of the vast array of stimuli that connect to a common reward motor. Presumably most activities can stimulate either the seeking or the liking submodules—depending on whether it is a question of expectations or actual execution.

Hedonism, or sensual pleasures, tends to be frowned upon in Western society. This sentiment may be explained by certain features of the pleasures typically associated with eudaemonia: They are either more lasting, less likely to cause harm by misuse, or considered virtuous and beneficial to society. Thus the preference for eudaemonic values may reflect an attempt to coach people towards choosing particular types of rewards. The preferred list would include those more likely to ensure optimal long-term happiness, and those favoured due to social or political priorities.

In short, although the neurobiology is shared, the sources of eudaemonic pleasures, and the way they are experienced, may differ appreciably from typical hedonic sensations; as may the long-term consequences of engaging in these two types of positive feelings. Consequently, the dichotomy may be warranted.

There is another aspect to the design of the brain that may help explain why people tend to consider eudaemonia as a different form of happiness.

In the absence of adverse factors, humans (as do other mammals) are apparently designed to be in a good mood—what I refer to as a default state of contentment (Grinde 2004). It is presumably in the interest of the genes to reside in a body/mind with a positive attitude to life, as this state of affair is conductive to the pursuits required for survival and procreation. The individual is more likely to take the trouble of looking for food or a spouse if in an agreeable mood. In support of the default contentment hypothesis, there is considerable data suggesting that people tend to be somewhat on the happy, optimistic and overconfident side of neutral (Diener and

Source of happiness		Hdoniae	Eudaimonia
Default contentment			+++
Sensual pleasures	Food	+++	+
	Drugs-alcohol	++	
	Sex	+++	+
Social relations	Falling in love		+++
	Old love		+++
	Parental love		+++
	Empathy		++
	Friendship		++
	Schadenfreude	+	
	Grief		+
Others	Meaning of life		++
	Engagement		++
	Religion	+	++
	Being in nature		+

Fig. 3.5 Attribution of various sources of happiness to either hedonia or eudaemonia. The number of + suggests relative potency based on a subjective evaluation. The table is solely meant to illustrate principles

Diener 1996; Lykken 2000; Johnson and Fowler 2011). The point is reflected in the tendency to gamble, in reporting more positive than negative feelings, as well as in personal assessment of happiness: When asked about subjective well-being, people claim, on the average, to be on the happy side (above five on a scale from 0 to10).

The default contentment is likely to be associated with eudaemonia rather than hedonia, as it does not require any external (sensual) stimuli, and as it is not in any way detrimental. Furthermore, retaining this state of mind is probably more important for the level of happiness compared to pursuing typical hedonic pleasures. Hedonic stimuli are generally fleeting, and sometimes at odds with long-term happiness, while a positive default state implies a continuous and wholesome source of bliss. Yet, it seems likely that the default contentment simply reflects that the mood modules are designed to operate with a net positive value as long as the negative modules are not specifically engaged.

The main point is that the reward (and punishment) modules may be activated in a number of ways, and that certain forms of activation are more likely to be labelled as hedonic, while others are considered eudaemonic (Fig. 3.5).

3.5 Individual Variations in Happiness

The discussion so far has focused on happiness in humans as a species. The biological approach is generally concerned primarily with species specific features, and to a less extent with the variations between individual members. The variation is, however, important; and can be addressed within the scope of a biological model.

In biology one distinguishes between *genotype* and *phenotype*; where the former is the particular genetic constitution of an individual, while the phenotype is the final product; that is, the qualities and personality of the person. The environment shapes the phenotype in conjunction with the genes.

Compared to most mammals, humans are genetically rather homogeneous due to our relatively recent common ancestor (dating back 150-200,000 years) (Garrigan et al. 2007; Green et al. 2010). (Not counting presumed minor genetic mixing with Neanderthals and Denisovans (Patterson et al. 2011), two human subspecies that split with our ancestors some 500,000 years ago.) Yet, as we presumably are designed to be moulded by the environment to a larger extent than other animals, there is considerable variability in phenotype.

The pursuit of happiness is about improving the phenotype towards more net positive activity in the mood modules. It is, for all practical purposes, not possible to change the genetic component; thus the focus should be on the environment. In order to make people happier, we need to adjust the environment (the way we live)—a topic I shall return to in later chapters.

In order to improve the environment we need to know what is desirable, but it is also useful to know what can potentially be achieved. If the level of happiness is primarily due to genetic factors, there is not much that can be done, while to the extent that the environment is important we can have an impact. In other words, we ought to know something about the heritability and genetics of happiness.

There are two main approaches aimed at evaluating genetic variation associated with a particular phenotypic trait: to estimate heritability and to look for specific genetic differences.

The easier part is to assess the heritability. Heritability is a measure for how much of the variation between individuals is caused by genes and how much by the environment. The question is normally investigated by examining individuals with various degrees of shared genetic and environmental background—such as identical twins and other siblings—preferably including both persons reared together and reared apart.

In order to arrive at a score for heritability, one needs a reliable way to measure the feature in question. In the case of happiness, this is typically cared for by questionnaires of the type that ask people how well they feel. The results can be compounded to a happiness score and the score then evaluated as to what extent it correlates when comparing genetically closely related individuals (such as monozygotic twins) with less related individuals (such as dizygotic twins) (Fig. 3.6). In the case of monozygotic twins, the dots are more centred along the diagonal. Note also that the dots cluster in the upper right corner, implying that most subjects report happiness well above the middle value of 5.

The simplified version of estimating heritability is to start by finding the correlation factor (the degree of similarity) for happiness in, respectively, monozygotic and dizygotic twins. The difference between these two numbers is then multiplied by 2. For example, if the correlation factors are, respectively, between 0.5 and 0.3, then the heritability is $(0.5–0.3) \times 2 = 0.4$. This means that 40% of the variation observed is expected to be due to variation in genes; and conversely, 60% due to the environment.

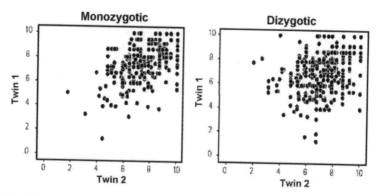

Fig. 3.6 Twin correlation in response to questionnaires assessing subjective well-being (on a scale from 0 to 10). In the *left* panel monozygotic, in the *right* dizygotic twins. Each dot represents one twin couple. The figure is kindly provided by RB Nes, the underlying data are published in (Nes et al. 2006)

Heritability measures should, however, be interpreted with caution. There are two main concerns. For one, the results are only valid for the population in question. If the population happens to have a homogeneous environment (as it relates to the particular trait), the heritability score will be elevated, simply because in this case the environment contributes less. Even twins reared apart typically grow up in relatively similar environments, such as middle class Western culture. Industrialised countries only span a small part of the possible environmental variability available for humans. The relative similarity in environment implies that the estimated heritability is somewhat high; that is, a more varied environment would have yielded a stronger environmental effect. The second problem is whether the method used for assessing the trait (in this case, questionnaires), really offers a measure of happiness; an issue discussed in Sect. 1.4. These caveats should be kept in mind when discussing the heritability of happiness.

When examining subjective well-being, it is typically found that the heritability is in the order of 30–40% (Tellegen et al. 1988; Lykken and Tellegen 1996). Looking more broadly at life quality, rather than just well-being, heritability estimates of 36–50% have been published (Nes et al. 2006; Bartels and Boomsma 2009; Bartels et al. 2010; Schnittker 2008). The heritability of negative emotions, such as depression and neuroticism, are in a similar range (Sullivan et al. 2000; Boardman et al. 2008). 'Subjective wellbeing' (as assessed by caretakers) has been found to be equally heritable in chimpanzees as well (Weiss et al. 2002).

It may be added that most mental traits examined tend to end up with a heritability scores between 30 and 70%. Thus, the propensity for happiness depends about as much on genetic constitution as, for example, the propensity for intelligence and anger.

Much of the daily conscious activity has only limited relevance for the level of happiness. People do not experience life as a stream of either good or bad events, but rather as a relatively steady state. Mood may move slightly up or down, as when respectively working on an interesting task or feeling bored; and, more rarely, episodes may cause a particular surge of pleasure or pain. In other words, the mood modules do not normally dominate the mind, but that does not imply they are inactive. It seems more appropriate to envision a tonus of mood caused by a balance of positive and negative activity.

The steady-state tonus presumably reflects what some scientists refers to as a *setpoint of happiness* (Lykken 2000). Particular events may move a person up or down relative to the baseline, but the baseline itself is primarily a consequence of genetic factors and previous experiences (i.e. the environment). While it may be easy to find a stimulus that sends happiness temporarily beyond the baseline; it is more difficult, but not impossible, to boost the baseline itself.

Apparently, most of the specific events that happen to us have only temporary effects on happiness. Within 3 months of even rather drastic incidents, such as breaking a leg or winning the lottery, we tend to return to pretty much the same level (Suh et al. 1996). On the other hand, over longer periods, such as 6–10 years, longitudinal studies of well-being in twins indicate only 50% stability of score (Nes et al. 2006; Lykken and Tellegen 1996; Johnson et al. 2005). Thus the effect of the environment, and how we choose to deal with the quandaries of life, may move us slowly towards a different set point.

The exception to the above rule is the occurrence of drastic, *unfortunate* changes in life situation, such as the loss of work (Lucas et al. 2004) or partner (Lucas et al. 2003). It seems that people are less influenced by positive incidents— the elevation of happiness tends to be short term. This observation is presumably related to the notion that negative experiences are associated with more intense and lasting emotional reactions than positive experiences (Fredrickson and Losada 2005), presumably because a single threat can have a far more drastic effect on genetic fitness (e.g., leading to death), than can a single fortunate event.

While women have on the average approximately the same score of happiness as do men, they report significantly more negative emotions (Nes et al. 2006, 2007; Michaelson et al. 2009). This apparent discrepancy may be due to women being both more vulnerable to negative affect, but also more able to cope and retain a high spirit. In other words, the normal distribution of well-being may have a wider base (a higher variance) in the case of women compared to men.

Heritability studies can be used to estimate the general importance of genes versus environment; they cannot, however, tell whether the level or happiness in one particular individual is due to the genes or to how that person was raised (Fig. 3.7).

Genetic studies, particularly with the advent of recent improvements in molecular biology, can help pinpoint the genes involved in causing heritability; and consequently offer a way of assessing the genetic disposition of an individual. However, as in the case of other complex traits, it has proven exceedingly difficult to identify the genes responsible for the variation in happiness.

The starting point for this kind of endeavour is typically to do *genome wide association studies*. Genetic markers (for example, in the form of point mutations) spread out along the entire human genome are examined to see if any of them

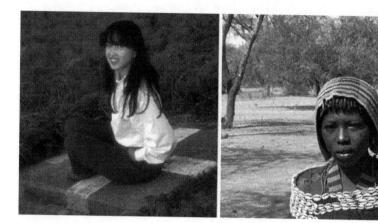

Fig. 3.7 Is it the environment or the genes that cause differences in happiness? Research suggests that within a typical, industrialised society the genes are responsible for 30–40% of the variation. It is, however, difficult to compare different cultures—not the least due to the problem of translating the questionnaires used to assess wellbeing. It is even more difficult to differentiate between nature and nurture when considering the happiness set point of an individual. (Photo: B. Grinde)

correlate with the trait in question. The results may pinpoint putative gene regions that account for part of the heritability.

In the case of happiness, at least one such study has been reported (Bartels et al. 2010). Not surprisingly, they did not find any obvious association between subjective well-being and regions of the genome. They did report a weak linkage between the trait and two regions, one at the end of the long arm of chromosome 19 and the other at the short arm of chromosome 1, but neither score had a high statistical significance. Based on the experience with similar weak links in studies of other traits (such as various mental and somatic disorders), the results may not be reproducible.

The likely conclusion is that the heritability of subjective wellbeing cannot be delegated to a few genes. The propensity for happiness is more likely due to the combination of particular versions of a large subset of genes.

It should be mentioned that *rare* genetic mutations, such as those causing any serious disease, may impact on happiness; either directly or indirectly (due to the debilitating nature of the disease). For example, even prodromal cases of Huntington disease have an elevated level of depression and suicidal behaviour (Fiedorowicz et al. 2011). Rare mutations, however, are unlikely to be detected in genome wide association studies.

The human brain has a complex genetic expression profile, utilising a majority of the 21,000 protein encoding genes of the human genome (Ramskold et al. 2009). The conclusion that the balanced effect of a large variety of genes is responsible for a trait such as well-being is therefore not surprising. Yet, the negative result of the association study does not imply that we cannot locate relevant genes by other methods.

The serotonin transporter gene (SLC6A4) is a possible candidate. The protein produced by this gene transport the neurotransmitter serotonin back into the cells, thereby having an effect on the transmission of signal between nerve cells employing serotonin. Serotonin is a key neurotransmitter associated with mood. It is best known through the effect of anti-depressive medicine, such as Prozac, that boosts the activity of serotonin in the brain.

There are two main versions of the genetic region that regulates the production of the serotonin transporter: The long version causes a higher level of the transporter than the short version. People with only the long version are reportedly twice as likely to say they are satisfied with life (De Neve 2011). Moreover, the less active version has been associated with increased risk of developing depression when exposed to unfortunate circumstances of life (Karg et al. 2011). Although both versions of this gene are reasonably common, the association to well-being was apparently lost in the genome wide association study mentioned above, and the effects have been questioned (Duncan and Keller 2011).

The main points in this chapter are:

1. All bodily components are vulnerable to malfunction (evolution does not create perfect organs or species), but the brain is particularly vulnerable.
2. If the environment is different from what the genes are designed to live in, the risk of ailments increases.
3. The mood modules are responsible for generating affect. There are three core modules: seeking, liking (for reward) and pain (for punishment).
4. It is difficult to predict whether a situation, or a type of emotion, activates pleasure or pain. Fear and grief, for example, can activate either—depending primarily on cognitive input.
5. The mood modules operate on a principle of 'common currency'. The concepts of anhedonia, pleasure related analgesia and alliesthesia reflect this observation.
6. We have some ideas as to the neurobiology involved.
7. The three core modules apparently cater to all sorts of positive and negative feelings—hedonic and eudaemonic pleasures have a shared neurobiology.
8. If negative feelings are not activated, people tend to be above 'neutral' on a happiness scale—a notion referred to as a default state of contentment.
9. Eudaemonia relates to the default contentment, as well as to pleasures considered healthy (less likely to be misused), more lasting, virtuous and good for society.
10. Each person appears to have a set point of happiness.
11. Although individual genetic constitution is important for happiness, there is considerable room for improvement by optimising the environment.

References

Ashby, F. G., Isen, A. M., & Turken, A. U. (1999). A neuropsychological theory of positive affect and its influence on cognition. *Psychological Review, 106*, 529–550.

Barbano, M. F., & Cador, M. (2007). Opioids for hedonic experience and dopamine to get ready for it. *Psychopharmacology (Berl), 191*, 497–506.

Bartels, M., & Boomsma, D. I. (2009). Born to be happy? The etiology of subjective well-being. *Behavior Genetics, 39*, 605–615.

Bartels, M., Saviouk, V., de Moor, M. H., Willemsen, G., van Beijsterveldt, T. C., Hottenga, J. J., et al. (2010). Heritability and genome-wide linkage scan of subjective happiness. *Twin Research and Human Genetics, 13*, 135–142.

Berna, C., Leknes, S., Holmes, E. A., Edwards, R. R., Goodwin, G. M., & Tracey, I. (2010). Induction of depressed mood disrupts emotion regulation neurocircuitry and enhances pain unpleasantness. *Biological Psychiatry, 67*, 1083–1090.

Berridge, K. C. (2003). Pleasures of the brain. *Brain and Cognition, 52*, 106–128.

Blood, A. J., & Zatorre, R. J. (2001). Intensely pleasurable responses to music correlate with activity in brain regions implicated in reward and emotion. *Proceedings of the National Academy of Sciences U S A, 98*, 11818–11823.

Boardman, J. D., Blalock, C. L., & Button, T. M. (2008). Sex differences in the heritability of resilience. *Twin Research and Human Genetics, 11*, 12–27.

Cabanac, M. (1979). Sensory pleasure. *The Quarterly Review of Biology, 54*, 1–29.

Chase DL, Koelle MR (2007) Biogenic amine neurotransmitters in C. elegans. *WormBook*, 1–15.

Craig, A. D. (2003). A new view of pain as a homeostatic emotion. *Trends in Neurosciences, 26*, 303–307.

De Neve, J. E. (2011). Functional polymorphism (5-HTTLPR) in the serotonin transporter gene is associated with subjective well-being: Evidence from a US nationally representative sample. *Journal of Human Genetics, 56*, 456–459.

Diener, E., & Diener, C. (1996). Most people are happy. *Psychological Science, 7*, 181–185.

Duncan, L. E., & Keller, M. C. (2011). A critical review of the first 10 years of candidate gene-by-environment interaction research in psychiatry. *American Journal of Psychiatry, 168*, 1041–1049.

Eisenberger, N. I., Lieberman, M. D., & Williams, K. D. (2003). Does rejection hurt? An fMRI study of social exclusion. *Science, 302*, 290–292.

Fiedorowicz, J. G., Mills, J. A., Ruggle, A., Langbehn, D., & Paulsen, J. S. (2011). Suicidal behavior in prodromal Huntington disease. *Neurodegenerative Diseases Journal, 8*, 483–490.

Fields, H. L. (2007). Understanding how opioids contribute to reward and analgesia. *Regional Anesthesia and Pain Medicine, 32*, 242–246.

Forsberg, G., Wiesenfeld-Hallin, Z., Eneroth, P., & Sodersten, P. (1987). Sexual behavior induces naloxone-reversible hypoalgesia in male rats. *Neuroscience Letters, 81*, 151–154.

Fredrickson, B. L. (1998). What good are positive emotions? *Review of General Psychology, 2*, 300–319.

Fredrickson, B. L., & Losada, M. F. (2005). Positive affect and the complex dynamics of human flourishing. *American Psychologist, 60*, 678–686.

Garrigan, D., Kingan, S. B., Pilkington, M. M., Wilder, J. A., Cox, M. P., Soodyall, H., et al. (2007). Inferring human population sizes, divergence times and rates of gene flow from mitochondrial, X and Y chromosome resequencing data. *Genetics, 177*, 2195–2207.

Gorwood, P. (2008). Neurobiological mechanisms of anhedonia. *Dialogues in Clinical Neuroscience, 10*, 291–299.

Green, R. E., Krause, J., Briggs, A. W., Maricic, T., Stenzel, U., Kircher, M., et al. (2010). A draft sequence of the Neandertal genome. *Science, 328*, 710–722.

Grinde, B. (2004). Can the evolutionary perspective on well-being help us improve society? *World Futures, 60*, 317–329.

Grinde, B., & Patil, G. G. (2009). Biophilia: Does visual contact with nature impact on health and well-being? *International Journal of Environmental Research and Public Health, 6*, 2332–2343.

Izuma, K., Saito, D. N., & Sadato, N. (2008). Processing of social and monetary rewards in the human striatum. *Neuron, 58*, 284–294.

Izuma, K., Saito, D. N., & Sadato, N. (2010). Processing of the incentive for social approval in the ventral striatum DURING charitable donation. *Journal of Cognitive Neuroscience, 22*, 621–631.

Johnson, D. D., & Fowler, J. H. (2011). The evolution of overconfidence. *Nature, 477*, 317–320.

Johnson, W., McGue, M., & Krueger, R. F. (2005). Personality stability in late adulthood: A behavioral genetic analysis. *Journal of Personality, 73*, 523–552.

Karg, K., Burmeister, M., Shedden, K., & Sen, S. (2011). The serotonin transporter promoter variant (5-HTTLPR), stress, and depression meta-analysis revisited: Evidence of genetic moderation. *Archives of General Psychiatry, 68*, 444–454.

Kringelbach, M. L., & Berridge, K. C. (2009). Towards a functional neuroanatomy of pleasure and happiness. *Trends in Cognitive Sciences, 13*, 479–487.

Kringelbach, M., & Berridge, K. (2010). *Pleasures of the brain*. Oxford: Oxford University Press.

Leknes, S., Lee, M., Berna, C., Andersson, J., & Tracey, I. (2011). Relief as a reward: Hedonic and neural responses to safety from pain. *PLoS ONE, 6*, e17870.

Leknes, S., & Tracey, I. (2008). A common neurobiology for pain and pleasure. *Nature Reviews Neuroscience, 9*, 314–320.

Lieberman, M. D., & Eisenberger, N. I. (2009). Neuroscience pains and pleasures of social life. *Science, 323*, 890–891.

Lucas, R. E., Clark, A. E., Georgellis, Y., & Diener, E. (2003). Reexamining adaptation and the set point model of happiness: Reactions to changes in marital status. *Journal of Personality and Social Psychology, 84*, 527–539.

Lucas, R. E., Clark, A. E., Georgellis, Y., & Diener, E. (2004). Unemployment alters the set point for life satisfaction. *Psychological Science, 15*, 8–13.

Lykken, D. (2000). *Happiness: The nature and nurture of joy and contentment*. New York: St. Martin's Griffin.

Lykken, D., & Tellegen, A. (1996). Happiness is a stochastic phenomenon. *Psychological Science, 7*, 186–189.

McWilliams, L. A., Goodwin, R. D., & Cox, B. J. (2004). Depression and anxiety associated with three pain conditions: Results from a nationally representative sample. *Pain, 111*, 77–83.

Michaelson, J., Abdallah, S., Steuer, N., Thompson, S., & Marks, N. (2009). *National accounts of well-being: Bringing real wealth onto the balance sheet*. London: New Economic Foundation.

Miller, J. M., Vorel, S. R., Tranguch, A. J., Kenny, E. T., Mazzoni, P., van Gorp, W. G., et al. (2006). Anhedonia after a selective bilateral lesion of the globus pallidus. *American Journal of Psychiatry, 163*, 786–788.

Moffitt, T. E., Caspi, A., Taylor, A., Kokaua, J., Milne, B. J., Polanczyk, G., et al. (2010). How common are common mental disorders? Evidence that lifetime prevalence rates are doubled by prospective versus retrospective ascertainment. *Psychological Medicine, 40*, 899–909.

Narita, M., Kishimoto, Y., Ise, Y., Yajima, Y., Misawa, K., & Suzuki, T. (2005). Direct evidence for the involvement of the mesolimbic kappa-opioid system in the morphine-induced rewarding effect under an inflammatory pain-like state. *Neuropsychopharmacology, 30*, 111–118.

Nes, R. B., Roysamb, E., Reichborn-Kjennerud, T., Harris, J. R., & Tambs, K. (2007). Symptoms of anxiety and depression in young adults: Genetic and environmental influences on stability and change. *Twin Research and Human Genetics, 10*, 450–461.

Nes, R. B., Roysamb, E., Tambs, K., Harris, J. R., & Reichborn-Kjennerud, T. (2006). Subjective well-being: Genetic and environmental contributions to stability and change. *Psychological Medicine, 36*, 1033–1042.

Nesse, R. M. (2004). Natural selection and the elusiveness of happiness. *Philosophical Transactions of the Royal Society of London. Series B, Biological sciences, 359*, 1333–1347.

Nieto-Fernandez, F., Andrieux, S., Idrees, S., Bagnall, C., Pryor, S. C., & Sood, R. (2009). The effect of opioids and their antagonists on the nocifensive response of Caenorhabditis elegans to noxious thermal stimuli. *Invertebrate Neuroscience, 9*, 195–200.

O'Connor, M. F., Wellisch, D. K., Stanton, A. L., Eisenberger, N. I., Irwin, M. R., & Lieberman, M. D. (2008). Craving love? Enduring grief activates brain's reward center. *Neuroimage, 42*, 969–972.

Panksepp, J. (1998). *Affective neuroscience*. New York: Oxford University Press.

Reich. D., Patterson, N., Kircher, M., Delfin, F., Nandineni, M. R., Pugach, I., Ko, A. M., Ko, Y. C., Jinam, T. A., Phipps, M. E., Saitou, N., Wollstein, A., Kayser, M., Paabo, S., & Stoneking, M. (2011). Denisova admixture and the first modern human dispersals into Southeast Asia and Oceania. *American Journal of Human Genetics, 89*(4), 516–528.

Pecina, S. (2008). Opioid reward 'liking' and 'wanting' in the nucleus accumbens. *Physiology & Behavior, 94*, 675–680.

Petrovic, P., Dietrich, T., Fransson, P., Andersson, J., Carlsson, K., & Ingvar, M. (2005). Placebo in emotional processing—induced expectations of anxiety relief activate a generalized modulatory network. *Neuron, 46*, 957–969.

Price, D. D., Harkins, S. W., & Baker, C. (1987). Sensory-affective relationships among different types of clinical and experimental pain. *Pain, 28*, 297–307.

Ramskold, D., Wang, E. T., Burge, C. B., & Sandberg, R. (2009). An abundance of ubiquitously expressed genes revealed by tissue transcriptome sequence data. *PLoS Computational Biology, 5*, e1000598.

Reboucas, E. C., Segato, E. N., Kishi, R., Freitas, R. L., Savoldi, M., Morato, S., et al. (2005). Effect of the blockade of mu1-opioid and 5HT2A-serotonergic/alpha1-noradrenergic receptors on sweet-substance-induced analgesia. *Psychopharmacology (Berl), 179*, 349–355.

Roy, M., Peretz, I., & Rainville, P. (2008). Emotional valence contributes to music-induced analgesia. *Pain, 134*, 140–147.

Schlaepfer, T. E., Cohen, M. X., Frick, C., Kosel, M., Brodesser, D., Axmacher, N., et al. (2008). Deep brain stimulation to reward circuitry alleviates anhedonia in refractory major depression. *Neuropsychopharmacology, 33*, 368–377.

Schnittker, J. (2008). Happiness and success: Genes, families, and the psychological effects of socioeconomic position and social support. *American Journal of Science, 114*(Suppl), S233–S259.

Smith, K. S., & Berridge, K. C. (2007). Opioid limbic circuit for reward: Interaction between hedonic hotspots of nucleus accumbens and ventral pallidum. *Journal of Neuroscience, 27*, 1594–1605.

Stevenson, G. W., Bilsky, E. J., & Negus, S. S. (2006). Targeting pain-suppressed behaviors in preclinical assays of pain and analgesia: Effects of morphine on acetic acid-suppressed feeding in C57BL/6 J mice. *Journal of Pain, 7*, 408–416.

Stuber, G. D., Sparta, D. R., Stamatakis, A. M., van Leeuwen, W. A., Hardjoprajitno, J. E., Cho, S., et al. (2011). Excitatory transmission from the amygdala to nucleus accumbens facilitates reward seeking. *Nature, 475*, 377–380.

Suh, E., Diener, E., & Fujita, F. (1996). Events and subjective well-being: Only recent events matter. *Journal of Personality and Social Psychology, 70*, 1091–1102.

Sullivan, P. F., Neale, M. C., & Kendler, K. S. (2000). Genetic epidemiology of major depression: Review and meta-analysis. *American Journal of Psychiatry, 157*, 1552–1562.

Tabibnia, G., & Lieberman, M. D. (2007). Fairness and cooperation are rewarding: Evidence from social cognitive neuroscience. *Social Cognitive Neuroscience of Organizations, 1118*, 90–101.

Tabibnia, G., Satpute, A. B., & Lieberman, M. D. (2008). The sunny side of fairness: Preference for fairness activates reward circuitry (and disregarding unfairness activates self-control circuitry). *Psychological Science, 19*, 339–347.

Takahashi, H., Kato, M., Matsuura, M., Mobbs, D., Suhara, T., & Okubo, Y. (2009). When your gain is my pain and your pain is my gain: Neural correlates of envy and schadenfreude. *Science, 323*, 937–939.

Tamietto, M., & de, G. B. (2010). Neural bases of the non-conscious perception of emotional signals. *Nature Reviews Neuroscience, 11*, 697–709.

Tellegen, A., Lykken, D. T., Bouchard, T. J, Jr, Wilcox, K. J., Segal, N. L., & Rich, S. (1988). Personality similarity in twins reared apart and together. *Journal of Personality and Social Psychology, 54*, 1031–1039.

Villemure, C., Slotnick, B. M., & Bushnell, M. C. (2003). Effects of odors on pain perception: Deciphering the roles of emotion and attention. *Pain, 106*, 101–108.

Watson, K. K., & Platt, M. L. (2008). Neuroethology of reward and decision making. *Philosophical Transactions of the Royal Society of London. Series B, Biological sciences, 363*, 3825–3835.

Weiss, A., King, J. E., & Enns, R. M. (2002). Subjective well-being is heritable and genetically correlated with dominance in chimpanzees (Pan troglodytes). *Journal of Personality and Social Psychology, 83*, 1141–1149.

Wittchen, H. U., Jacobi, F., Rehm, J., Gustavsson, A., Svensson, M., Jonsson, B., et al. (2011). The size and burden of mental disorders and other disorders of the brain in Europe 2010. *European Neuropsychopharmacology, 21*, 655–679.

Chapter 4
Mental Health

Abstract Mental disorders are arguably the biggest health problems in industrialised societies. The innate tendency to develop a particular ailment is expected to approximate normal distribution, a discord environment moves the phenotype curve in the direction of higher prevalence. The most prevalent mental problems are associated with unwarranted activity in three punishment submodules—pain, fear and low mood—causing, respectively, chronic pain, anxiety and depression. These defence modules are particularly relevant as to mental health because they activate negative feelings and are easily triggered. Conversely, hyperactivity in reward modules is rarely a problem. Discords are mismatches— between the human environment of evolutionary adaptation and present life—that can have negative consequences for health and happiness. The concept of Darwinian happiness is based on the dual principle of avoiding discords and boosting the positive output of mood modules.

Keywords Mental disorders · DALY · Anxiety · Depression · Low mood · Pain · Defence functions · Discords · Stress · Environment of evolutionary adaptation

4.1 The Link Between Happiness and Mental Disorders

Mental disorders have become a major burden in industrialised societies; in terms of the quality of life of citizens, and by disrupting the economy as a common cause of sick leaves and disability. As previously mentioned, the statistics suggest that mental dysfunction is perhaps the number one health problem. It accounts for more than a fourth of the total morbidity burden (in terms of disability-adjusted life years—DALYs); and it is estimated that as much as half the population will suffer from a diagnosable condition at some point in life, while a third suffers in any

B. Grinde, *The Biology of Happiness*, SpringerBriefs in Well-Being and Quality of Life Research, DOI: 10.1007/978-94-007-4393-9_4, © The Author(s) 2012

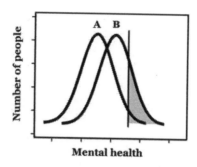

Fig. 4.1 The disposition to develop mental problems, e.g. in the form of anxiety and depression, is presumably distributed in the population in a way that approximates a normal distribution (curve A). If the environment is not optimal, the actual burden of disease will increase—as suggested by moving the distribution of mental health from A ('neutral'—no particular effect of the environment) to B (suboptimal environment). Given that problems above a certain threshold (vertical line) are considered a mental disorder, the fraction of the population suffering will increase—as suggested by the *grey area* under the two curves

given year (Moffitt et al. 2010; Wittchen et al. 2011). These figures do not include problems such as chronic pain or common neurological disorders such as stroke, Parkinson's disease and multiple sclerosis.

Mental health has consequently received increasing attention from authorities. The present model of happiness suggests an explanation for the predicament, and points towards possible strategies for redemption.

It seems unlikely that the current statistics of mental problems reflect the natural state of the human mind. The most common conditions, such as anxiety and depression, would be expected to be under considerable negative selection in a tribal, hunter-gatherer setting—at least the more pathological forms. A reasonable interpretation is that the high prevalence is due to suboptimal aspects of the present environment.

Some individuals are genetically more prone than others to develop psychiatric conditions. Those with a distinct genetic disadvantage would probably get sick regardless of the environment, but an unfavourable environment will lower the cut-off (as to the genetic disposition required), causing a larger fraction of the population to develop disorders. In Fig. 4.1, curve A represents the genotype, which in a 'neutral' environment is centred on the same value as the phenotype, while curve B indicates the phenotype in an environment causing an increase in mental problems. (Curves are given a normal distribution for simplicity; the distribution of symptoms (B) tends to have a longer tail to the right.)

There are two main quandaries associated with mental problems: One, patients are unhappy, i.e. their quality of life suffers; and two, the patients do not function in society, which indirectly may, or may not cause further suffering.

The two problems do not necessarily go together. Intellectually disabled people, for example, may be happy as long as they are cared for (Robinson 2000; Williams et al. 2006); while a depressed person can be deeply unhappy, but still function satisfactorily.

The unhappiness part of the problem is (in the present terminology) due to unfortunate activity in the mood modules—typically due to activation of the punishment module. The two most common types of mental disorders, those related to anxiety and depression, can be ascribed to malfunctioning of particular submodules engaged in negative feelings.

Adverse events—such as hunger, fear or breaking a leg—cause negative feelings that temporarily reverse the default state of contentment, but the brain normally returns to a positive frame once the particular experience is ended. It is in the interest of the genes not to prolong the pain beyond what is useful: The pain should teach you to avoid similar situations in the future, and (if relevant) help protect the wounded part from further damage. The unhappiness aspect of mental illness reflects either a negative reaction in excess of what is (biologically) appropriate or the preservation of discontent in the absence of adverse events. In both cases it is a question of distorted functioning of neural networks associated with the punishment submodules.

The submodules most frequently involved in a declining happiness are: *fear*, *low mood* and *pain*. Distorted functioning of these three can be referred to as, respectively, anxiety, depression and non-functional (chronic) pain. Perhaps not surprisingly, these submodules appear to be the ones most vulnerable to distortion in an industrialised society. Their presumed related neurobiology (the punishment module), may contribute to the comorbidity observed (Berna et al. 2010; Kessler et al. 2005; McWilliams et al. 2004).

Even a subclinical level of unwarranted activity in these modules would be expected to reduce happiness—exemplified by an undue rumination on worries or a vague gloom—thus the diagnosable psychiatric disorders may be the tip of the iceberg as to reduced quality of life caused by distorted functioning. Moreover, conditions often diagnosed in other terms may, to a large extent, be a consequence of problems with these three submodules. Sleep problems are, for example, often related to anxiety; while drug abuse is related to low mood. As expected, psychological indicators suggest that a tendency towards anxiety or depression correlates negatively with positive affect and subjective well-being (Nes et al. 2007; Watson and Naragon-Gainey 2010).

The role of the three submodules as to mental health will be discussed briefly.

Pain is the classical example of a punishing sensation. When called for, pain is an important and highly appropriate response. In fact, a rare genetic condition causes the 'sufferer' to be unable to experience pain (Cox et al. 2006). These people, with congenital insensitivity to pain, usually die young due to an inability to avoid harming the body. Simply sitting still on a chair can be damaging if you do not feel the discomfort caused by lack of movement. The blood supply to the part you rest your weight on will eventually become too limited to maintain oxygen balance—cells will die and necrosis will follow. When feeling discomfort, you shift position regularly and thereby avoid the problem. Consequently, it is not desirable to have no pain, the problem is inappropriate pain. Pain that lingers long after the reaction should have ended, or pain that is instigated in the absence of any cause, such as the phantom pain of an amputated limb (Giummarra et al. 2007).

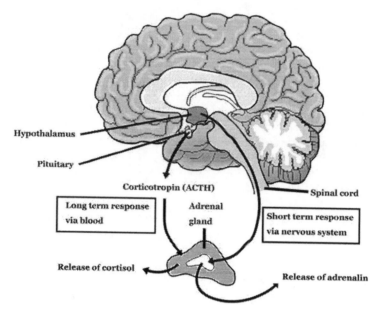

Fig. 4.2 The fear function is a coordinated response to dangerous situations. It is initiated in the brain, but to a large extent conducted by endocrine organs, particularly the adrenal gland. The first (short-term) step is when nerve signals cause the adrenal gland to release adrenalin (epinephrine), a slightly slower step (long-term) involves signals passing from the hypothalamus to the pituitary, where the release of the hormone corticotrophin results in adrenal release of glucocorticoids such as cortisol. Adrenalin and cortisol regulate various functions around the body with the effect of making the individual ready for fight-or-flight. Frequent activation of the function can cause stress symptoms and/or anxiety

Inappropriate pain is a major problem in Western societies. Some 20% of the adult European population suffers from chronic pain (Breivik et al. 2006); the majority of cases are likely to be inappropriate. The pain is often associated with muscle and skeletal problems, and/or with misplaced activity of the immune system. Rheumatic diseases are examples of the latter.

Anxiety may be regarded as perverted activity of the fear submodule (Fig. 4.2). This module is of considerable importance in evolutionary terms, and has a reasonably well-characterised neurobiology that overlaps with regions involved with the more classical forms of pain, for example, in the amygdala and periaqueductal grey (Bandler and Shipley 1994; Panksepp 1998). The main function of fear is, like pain, to avoid hurting or endangering oneself, which explains the connection with the punishment module. It is estimated that some 15–20% of the population suffer from anxiety related disorders (Moffitt et al. 2010; Wittchen et al. 2011).

As in the case of pain, a total lack of fear can be dangerous. A woman who lost her capacity to experience fear due to damage to the amygdala, stopped avoiding risk behaviour, such as playing with snakes (Feinstein et al. 2011); and a loss of fear of height may cause a climber to take unnecessary risks and fall down.

It appears as if the amygdala is required to balanced fear and curiosity. If you are not afraid, you approach objects and situations for the purpose of learning.

Depression is, in the present terminology, associated with hyperactivity of a 'low mood' module. While fear has an obvious biological function, it is less clear why we need a module for low mood.

One likely purpose is to secure social relations. In the Stone Age a lack of a strong social network would be a serious threat to survival. The low mood induces a negative feeling (loneliness) in order to teach the individual to seek companionship with others. A connection between the neurobiology of pain and that of social rejection has been documented (Eisenberger et al. 2003).

The low-mood module is probably also activated when unsuccessful in a task, such as missing the game in a hunt; or, these days, flunk an exam. Again the feeling induced ought to be unpleasant in order to teach the individual to try to avoid ending up in the same situation the next time; that is, to try a different strategy. Even the stimulation of the immune system caused by an infection may promote depression (Raison et al. 2010); possibly because contracting an infection is considered, in evolutionary terms, something one should learn to avoid. Clinical depression has a prevalence of some 10–20% (Moffitt et al. 2010; Wittchen et al. 2011).

Unwarranted activity in these three submodules tends to diminish rewarding sensations and demolish the default state of contentment. Preventing or treating these ailments is arguably the most compelling way of improving well-being—and mental health—in society.

It is not surprising that mental complaints are associated with undesirable activity in feelings perceived as negative. There is not the same cause for complaint if the reward circuits of the brain are hyperactive. Unfortunately, this is a less likely scenario. One may argue that the manic phase of dipolar disorder is an undesirable consequence of hyperactivity in reward modules, and as such an exception to the above statement. Yet, without the down period (which, per definition, is part of the disease), the manic phase would presumably not be a major problem.

Pain, fear and low mood are all part of the *defence functions* of the body. Their primary function is to guide you away from dangerous or unfortunate situations. As such, they are designed to connect with the punishment module in order to drive an escape, and to help you remember that the situation triggering the reaction is something you should avoid.

Their functional role implies that they have a low threshold for activation. (Mobbs et al. 2007). It is, for example, better to jump at the sight of a stick resembling a snake, than not to respond when approaching a real snake. The point being that it is better for survival, when faced with danger, to act too often than too late. The cost of not reacting may be death, while the cost of overreacting is minimal as far as survival and procreation go. The easy triggering and the key role in survival (the latter implies that pain is important to remember) explain why negative events have a stronger impact on subjective well-being compared to positive events, as discussed in Sect. 3.5.

As regards individual happiness, the touchy character of negative modules may not seem advantageous; but as pointed out before, evolution is not concerned with optimising happiness. Furthermore, whether the perspective is survival or well-being, the occasional bursts of pain, fear or low mood do not matter—the main problem is the more chronic, often non-functional activity. In the Stone Age, that sort of activation would presumably imply reduced biological fitness, and thus be selected against. The problem seems to be that we live in a very different environment.

These factors—the negative sensations, the easy triggering, and the lingering reaction—are what cause the punishment submodules to top the list of mental disorders. Unfortunately, the reward modules are less likely to have elevated activity because they are not designed to be triggered that easily. As I shall return to in Chap. 5, the present model suggests a way out of the problem.

4.2 Darwinian Happiness and the Concept of Discords

I have previously described an evolutionary perspective on happiness using the phrase *Darwinian Happiness* (Grinde 1996, 2002a, b). The primary purpose of this concept was to help people take advantage of biological insight when exploring options meant to improve happiness. In this section, I shall recapitulate the principles behind the concept, while in the next chapter I shall discuss practical ways of enhancing happiness.

The two main principles of Darwinian happiness can be referred to with the words *stress* and *rewards*. Briefly, the key ideas are:

1. To avoid stress by adjusting the conditions of life to our innate tendencies.
2. To utilise the potential for rewarding sensations; that is, to optimise the net output of the mood modules.

Although the two principles may sound straightforward, it is not at all obvious how to best take advantage of them.

To begin with, the first research on animals, as well as experience with farm, pet and zoo animals, have taught us that offering them inappropriate conditions can have detrimental effects (Crawford and Krebs 2008; Moberg and Mench 2000). When people first brought in wild animals for display in zoological gardens, they assumed that as long as the animals were fed and given shelter, they should be fine. Eventually the zookeepers realised that this was not the case; the animals would, for example, scratch themselves to bleeding and refuse to eat. The situation did improve when the zookeepers adjusted not only nutritional and physical aspects of the environment to the requirements of the species in question, but also offered the animals a chance to live in a more natural way. The clue was to care for their behavioural needs.

For example, it causes stress to isolate a baboon from its flock, but also to force several adults of the naturally solitary orangutans to live together. In both cases, you are serving the animals conditions that are not in tune with the behavioural biology of the species. The consequences are hence likely to be detrimental.

Stress, in the present terminology, is a factor that increases the chance of ending up with some sort of malfunctioning. It is a consequence of a suboptimal environment. The brain is the most vulnerable organ in the body, and as indicated in the previous section, a malfunctioning brain more often than not implies excess activity in the punishment module, and a concomitant decrease in life quality.

Today, the notion of adapting the environment as much as possible to the innate tendencies of a particular species is obvious for those caring for animals—but perhaps less obvious for those dealing with humans. The 'mental environment' of present Western societies may be the cause of the high prevalence of mental problems. That is to say, submodules of the brain malfunction because we do not live the way we are designed by evolution to live.

I here use the word stress for the detrimental effects of living under unnatural conditions, but I should emphasise that this use of the concept departs somewhat from its classical meaning, which is associated with the 'fight-or-flight' response. While the word 'stress' in other terminologies can be either a positive or negative experience, as suggested in the example of an adrenalin kick, the present use focuses on negative aspects—more in the sense of a mental or physical 'strain'.

The term *environment of evolutionary adaptation*, or EEA, is used for the kind of conditions the genes have evolved to live in (Crawford and Krebs 2008). It should, however, be mentioned that the genes were not shaped in one particular environment, but rather over millions of years of interaction with various conditions. The emotions, for example, did not suddenly appear in the Stone Age, but precursors entered the brains of our ancestral mammals a couple of hundred million years ago. Subsequent evolution, all the way up to modern humans, has modified our emotional set-up, but the alterations have had to comply with the limitations governing the process of evolution.

Another point worth mentioning is that at present humans are adapted to diverse environments. The Inuit of Greenland are fit for a climate different from that of African Bantus. These variations in climatic adaptation, however, do not matter much for the present discussion: The more significant features of the human EEA are not so much a question of the physical environment, but rather of the social fabric; and the genes that influence social inclinations presumably do not differ that much.

Rather than considering EEA as a particular type of Stone Age conditions, it may be pertinent to define it as the *best* natural environment (i.e. prior to farming and industrialisation). And although it is difficult to describe one particular 'ideal' setting, it is possible to suggest certain attributes of the environment that may make a difference. We are adapted to a set of more or less vaguely defined conditions; and life in the Stone Age should offer valuable clues—that is, if we are able to describe it. In other words, Stone Age life, going back to 10,000 years or more, presumably included features that might suggest possible improvements as to present society.

Near-sightedness offers an illustrative example of the possible detrimental effects of the non-EEA qualities of our present environment (Fig. 4.3). Young people living in tribal or poor rural communities rarely need eyeglasses: While

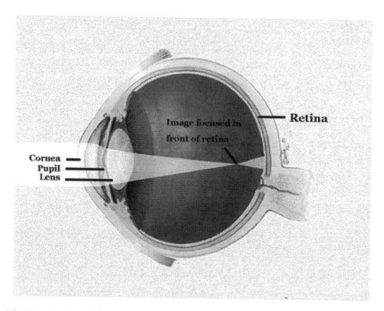

Fig. 4.3 Myopia (near-sightedness). For the eye to provide a picture in focus, the curvature of the lens must match the distance from the lens to the retina. The eyes develop as the child grows, but environmental factors (presumably in the form of visual impressions reaching the eye) will impact the process. If the environment differs from what the genes are adapted to, the lens may end up not matching the size of the eyeball. (Adapted from Wikimedia Commons, author: National Eye Institute.)

80% of the 18-year-old men of Singapore are near-sighted, only 1% of the rural population of Nepal has the same problem (Bock and Widdows 1990; Quinn et al. 1999). Environmental factors are the likely explanation for why so many individuals in industrialised societies suffer from myopia. At least three factors have been proposed:

1. The tendency to spend long periods of time focusing at fixed, close ranges, such as when reading.
2. The exposure to artificial light when the diurnal rhythm expects darkness; for example, in the form of keeping the lights on in the bedroom of children.
3. The lack of outdoor activities and the concomitant reduction in a variety of incoming visual signals.

The growth of both eyeballs and lenses is affected by light, and by how the eyes are used. Imperfections in this process may cause the focus to end up in front of the retina, which defines near-sightedness. Our genes are neither adapted to books nor to electricity. Yet, the evidence so far suggests that the more salient factor is the third one: Making sure the kids spend an hour or two outdoors everyday actually helps prevent near-sightedness (Rose et al. 2008).

The above example illustrates the possible consequences of having a lifestyle different from that for which our genes have prepared us. The genes have designed both physical features and mental functions to develop as we age, but correct maturation relies on appropriate external stimuli. While problems with the eyes are relatively easy to correct, mental disorders are a lot more difficult to alleviate. The important question is therefore whether we provide the emotional settings our genes are adapted to? Or does the stress associated with an environment at odds with the EEA cause imperfections in the development of mood modules, and a subsequent high prevalence of mental disorders?

It is well known from experiments with various animals that bringing up infants without proper maternal care, causes behavioural problems when the juveniles mature to adults. Humans are more versatile, yet most experts agree that similar gross deprivations cause problems in our species as well [for a discussion, see (Shonkoff and Phillips 2000)].

It should be pointed out that it is particularly detrimental to offer infants (and foetuses) inappropriate conditions, since this is the period in life with the most vigorous development, and as the effects of an inappropriate environment may have lasting consequences. In fact, as has been demonstrated in rodents, inappropriate care can affect not only the litter in question, but later generations as well by means of epigenetic changes (McGowan et al. 2011; Meaney and Ferguson-Smith 2010), as can maternal stress during pregnancy (Morgan and Bale 2011).

The example with myopia highlights two additional points:

1. It is difficult to predict which aspects of the environment are causative—research is required to choose among various conceivable explanations. Personally, I would have expected the first two factors mentioned in connection with myopia to be more important than the third, but empirical evidence suggests otherwise.
2. As suggested in Fig. 4.1, some people are more vulnerable to a less than optimal environment than others. Only those with a genetic susceptibility are likely to experience problems, whether in the form of myopia or anxiety. Yet, unfortunate aspects of the environment cause the fraction of sufferers to increase.

The differences between how we live and the life our genes are adapted to are commonly referred to as *mismatches* (Eaton et al. 1988). Mismatches may be associated with stress in the present meaning of the word, but more often they are not. For example, sleeping on a modern mattress is a mismatch, as these were not available in the Stone Age; yet to sleep on a mattress rather than on the ground most likely decreases your chance of developing back problems. It is a positive mismatch. I have used the word *discord* for situations where mismatches can have negative effects (Grinde 2002, 2009). Thus, while a mismatch can be entirely beneficial, a discord implies a situation that in most, or at least some people, causes an increased likelihood of developing medical problems, for example myopia or anxiety (Fig. 4.4).

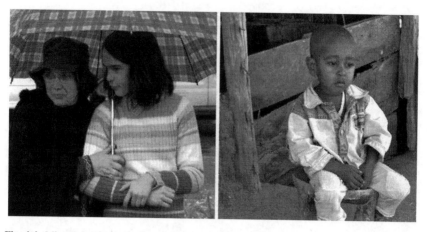

Fig. 4.4 Mismatches between the way we live and the life our genes prepare us for can be either advantageous, such as having an umbrella to shield from the rain; disadvantageous, such as being lonely due to the absence of social relations; or good for some people and bad for others. In cases where the effect is harmful, the mismatch is referred to as a discord. (Photo: B. Grinde)

A discord is defined as an adverse deviation from the EEA. Thus discord situations may have troubled our ancestors in the Stone Age as well, for example when a flood ruined the local environment, or when a child was orphaned.

Some mismatches may have both positive and negative consequences. The use of vaccines, for instance, has had a substantial positive effect on survival and health, yet we know that in certain people they cause serious side effects. For most people, however, the side effects are mild, and may be worth it—taking into consideration the protection afforded. Consequently, the line between mismatches and discords can be difficult to draw. It depends not only on an evaluation of positive and negative consequences, but also on the characteristics of the individual, and on personal preferences.

Another problem is that we are typically unaware of discord features in our environment—as exemplified by myopia. The cumulative effect of various discords may cause mental disease or decrease our quality of life, without anyone realising the reason for the distress.

In a majority of cases we know very little about what causes mental problems. Even if most of the discord situations have limited impact on most people, each type of situation may add a slight harm to a certain percentage, and all together be responsible for a lot of misery. In short, I find it unlikely that the prevalence of mental problems (or myopia) was as high in Stone Age communities as in present Western society, and the difference is presumably due to discord aspects of the way we live today.

Diet and physical activity represent aspects of life that have changed drastically since the Stone Age. We survive on a variety of food, and in the absence of exercise, yet it is well documented that modern 'junk' food and lack of physical

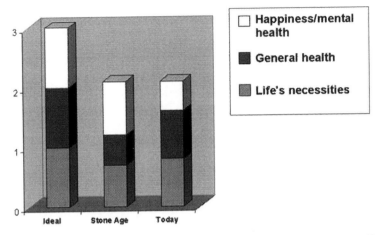

Fig. 4.5 Life quality in the Stone Age and today compared with the ideal situation. Three main factors that impact well-being—mental health, general health and life's necessities (in the meaning of food, shelter, safety, etc.)—are given the theoretical ideal value of one unit each. For the sake of illustration, the figure proposes that the sum was about the same then as now, but that we score better on general health while they scored better on mental health. As to life's necessities, some populations were probably troubled by lack of food then, as many people certainly are today

activity are discords reflected in their role in ailments such as diabetes and cardiovascular diseases. More recent evidence suggests that these discords are not just symptoms of mental problems, but can contribute as causative factors in mood disorders (Jacka et al. 2011; Pasco et al. 2011); implying a preventive potential in adapting the lifestyle.

The two principles Darwinian happiness is based on can be summarised as follows:

1. Living conditions should be adjusted to suit our inborn tendencies in order to avoid the stress brought on by a suboptimal environment. That is, one should strive to avoid discords, but not positive mismatches.
2. Agreeable sensations offered by the brain should be pursued while unpleasant sensations ought to be avoided. However, all types of positive experiences should be included, both hedonic and eudaemonic; and the aim should be to increase the output of the mood modules as integrated over a lifetime.

Darwinian happiness is a question of how successfully one follows these two principles. In order to employ the former, knowledge about the human EEA is important; for the latter, an understanding of how feelings are provided by the brain is relevant. The former is primarily about retaining the default state of contentment, and to avoid having a suboptimal environment trigger inappropriate activity in the punishment modules. The latter is about finding positive experiences, and learning to turn off the negative ones. It is consequently correct to state that both are about maximising output from the mood modules.

I do not claim that life was, on the average, better in the Stone Age. It seems likely that the people then had a somewhat lower prevalence of certain mental disorders, which today cause a considerable reduction of happiness—particularly anxiety and depression related conditions—but the Stone Agers were more likely to be troubled by other health problems due to the lack of modern medical care (Fig. 4.5).

The main points in this chapter are:

1. Mental disorders are arguably the biggest health problems in industrialised societies.
2. The tendency to develop a particular ailment may approximate normal distribution; a discord environment moves the phenotype curve towards a higher prevalence.
3. The most prevalent mental problems are associated with unwarranted activity in three punishment submodules—pain, fear, and low mood—causing respectively chronic pain, anxiety and depression.
4. These defence modules are particularly important for mental health because they activate negative feelings, are easily triggered and leave lasting impressions.
5. Hyperactivity in reward modules is rarely conceived as a problem.
6. Discords are mismatches—between the human environment of evolutionary adaptation and present life—that can have negative consequences for health and happiness.
7. The concept of Darwinian happiness is based on the dual principle of avoiding discords and boosting the positive output of mood modules.

References

Bandler, R., & Shipley, M. T. (1994). Columnar organization in the midbrain periaqueductal gray: Modules for emotional expression? *Trends in Neurosciences, 17*, 379–389.

Berna, C., Leknes, S., Holmes, E. A., Edwards, R. R., Goodwin, G. M., & Tracey, I. (2010). Induction of depressed mood disrupts emotion regulation neurocircuitry and enhances pain unpleasantness. *Biological Psychiatry, 67*, 1083–1090.

Bock, G., & Widdows, K. (1990). *Myopia and the control of eye growth.* New York: Ciba Foundation.

Breivik, H., Collett, B., Ventafridda, V., Cohen, R., & Gallacher, D. (2006). Survey of chronic pain in Europe: Prevalence, impact on daily life, and treatment. *European Journal of Pain, 10*, 287–333.

Cox, J. J., Reimann, F., Nicholas, A. K., Thornton, G., Roberts, E.,& Springell, K., et al. (2006). An SCN9A channelopathy causes congenital inability to experience pain. *Nature, 444*, 894–898.

Crawford, C., & Krebs, D. (2008). *Foundations of evolutionary psychology*. New York: Psychology Press.

Eaton, S. B., Konner, M., & Shostak, M. (1988). Stone agers in the fast lane: Chronic degenerative diseases in evolutionary perspective. *American Journal of Medicine, 84*, 739–749.

Eisenberger, N. I., Lieberman, M. D., & Williams, K. D. (2003). Does rejection hurt? An fMRI study of social exclusion. *Science, 302*, 290–292.

Feinstein, J. S., Adolphs, R., Damasio, A., & Tranel, D. (2011). The human amygdala and the induction and experience of fear. *Current Biology, 21*, 34–38.

Giummarra, M. J., Gibson, S. J., Georgiou-Karistianis, N., & Bradshaw, J. L. (2007). Central mechanisms in phantom limb perception: The past, present and future. *Brain Research Reviews, 54*, 219–232.

Grinde, B. (1996). Darwinian happiness: Biological advice on the quality of life. *Journal of Social and Evolutionary Systems, 19*, 31–40.

Grinde, B. (2002a). Happiness in the perspective of evolutionary psychology. *Journal of Happiness Studies, 3*, 331–354.

Grinde, B. (2002b). *Darwinian happiness - Evolution as a guide for living and understanding human behavior*. Princeton: The Darwin Press.

Grinde, B. (2009). Can the concept of discords help us find the causes of mental diseases? *Medical Hypotheses, 73*, 106–109.

Jacka, F. N., Kremer, P. J., Berk, M., de Silva-Sanigorski, A. M., Moodie, M., & Leslie, E. R., et al. (2011). A prospective study of diet quality and mental health in adolescents. *PLoS ONE, 6*, e24805.

Kessler, R. C., Chiu, W. T., Demler, O., Merikangas, K. R., & Walters, E. E. (2005). Prevalence, severity, and comorbidity of 12-month DSM-IV disorders in the National Comorbidity Survey Replication. *Archives of General Psychiatry, 62*, 617–627.

McGowan, P. O., Suderman, M., Sasaki, A., Huang, T. C., Hallett, M., Meaney, M. J., et al. (2011). Broad epigenetic signature of maternal care in the brain of adult rats. *PLoS ONE, 6*, e14739.

McWilliams, L. A., Goodwin, R. D., & Cox, B. J. (2004). Depression and anxiety associated with three pain conditions: Results from a nationally representative sample. *Pain, 111*, 77–83.

Meaney, M. J., & Ferguson-Smith, A. C. (2010). Epigenetic regulation of the neural transcriptome: The meaning of the marks. *Nature Neuroscience, 13*, 1313–1318.

Mobbs, D., Petrovic, P., Marchant, J. L., Hassabis, D., Weiskopf, N., & Seymour, B., et al. (2007). When fear is near: Threat imminence elicits prefrontal-periaqueductal gray shifts in humans. *Science, 317*, 1079–1083.

Moberg, G., & Mench, J. (2000). *The biology of animal stress*. Oxfordshire: CABI.

Moffitt, T. E., Caspi, A., Taylor, A., Kokaua, J., Milne, B. J., & Polanczyk, G., et al. (2010). How common are common mental disorders? Evidence that lifetime prevalence rates are doubled by prospective versus retrospective ascertainment. *Psychological Medicine, 40*, 899–909.

Morgan, C. P., & Bale, T. L. (2011). Early prenatal stress epigenetically programs dysmasculinization in second-generation offspring via the paternal lineage. *Journal of Neuroscience, 31*, 11748–11755.

Nes, R. B., Roysamb, E., Reichborn-Kjennerud, T., Harris, J. R., & Tambs, K. (2007). Symptoms of anxiety and depression in young adults: Genetic and environmental influences on stability and change. *Twin Research and Human Genetics, 10*, 450–461.

Panksepp, J. (1998). *Affective neruoscience*. New York: Oxford University Press.

Pasco, J. A., Jacka, F. N., Williams, L. J., Brennan, S. L., Leslie, E., & Berk, M. (2011). Don't worry, be active: Positive affect and habitual physical activity. *Australian and New Zealand Journal of Psychiatry, 45*, 1047–1052.

Quinn, G. E., Shin, C. H., Maguire, M. G., & Stone, R. A. (1999). Myopia and ambient lighting at night. *Nature, 399*, 113–114.

Robinson, R. (2000). Learning about happiness from persons with Down syndrome: Feeling the sense of joy and contentment. *American Journal Of Mental Retardation, 105*, 372–376.

Rose, K. A., Morgan, I. G., Ip, J., Kifley, A., Huynh, S., & Smith, W., et al. (2008). Outdoor activity reduces the prevalence of myopia in children. *Ophthalmology, 115*, 1279–1285.

Shonkoff, J., & Phillips, D. (2000). *From neurons to neighborhoods: The science of early childhood development*. Washington: National Academy Press.

Watson, D., & Naragon-Gainey, K. (2010). On the specificity of positive emotional dysfunction in psychopathology: Evidence from the mood and anxiety disorders and schizophrenia/ schizotypy. *Clinical Psychology Review, 30*, 839–848.

Williams, C. A., Beaudet, A. L., Clayton-Smith, J., Knoll, J. H., Kyllerman, M., & Laan, L. A., et al. (2006). Angelman syndrome 2005: Updated consensus for diagnostic criteria. *American Journal of Medical Genetics A, 140*, 413–418.

Wittchen, H. U., Jacobi, F., Rehm, J., Gustavsson, A., Svensson, M., & Jonsson, B., et al. (2011). The size and burden of mental disorders and other disorders of the brain in Europe 2010. *European Neuropsychopharmacology, 21*, 655–679.

Chapter 5
How to Improve Happiness

Abstract Most bodily functions can be exercised. In the case of brain functions, exercise typically results in a stronger module with more impact on the conscious self. One ought to avoid discords that cause exercise of the main punishment modules: fear, low mood and pain. The brain, however, contains both on and off 'switches' for the various mood modules. The training should be aimed at turning on positive feelings and off inappropriate negative feelings. Lack of proximity and skin contact between infants and parents are important discords regarding anxiety, a frail social network as well as failure in tasks are relevant discords in connection with depression, and lack of physical activity may contribute to pain. Meditative techniques may work as "exercise machines" for the mind. If happiness is the ultimate purpose, rationality is at times irrational.

Keywords Avoiding discords · Mental scar · Fear · Low mood · Brain exercise · Meditation · Rationalism · Religion · Smile · Laughter

5.1 Avoiding Discords

The default state of contentment implies an innate tendency to be in a good mood as long as there is no cause for negative feelings. It is presumably a characteristic feature of our species—as well as other mammals—but different individuals have a more or less strong innate disposition for contentment. As is the case for most traits, this disposition is expected to display a near normal distribution in the population.

The set point of happiness reflects the strength of innate dispositions for happiness, default contentment included, in combination with how the individual is shaped by the environment. Previous experiences, particularly in early life, can push the set point up or down on the scale from miserable to exultant. Unfortunately, as suggested in Chap. 4, in an environment troubled with discords, the set point is more likely to be pushed down.

A common misconception as to the idea of a 'setpoint' is that happiness cannot be improved. The level of affect (which, in the present terminology, means the net activity of the mood modules), may turn toward sadness or euphoria for periods, depending on important life events—such as respectively breaking a leg or winning a lottery—but the level tends to return to the normal value for the person in question relatively soon (Lykken 2000; Lucas 2008). If the best we can hope for is brief periods above our particular set point, is it worth the trouble to put a lot of effort into improving happiness?

As pointed out in Sect. 3.5, subjective well-being does change over the years. My stance is consequently that the effort towards improvement is worthwhile. Furthermore, it makes sense to focus on early life, the main period of brain development. Childhood experiences may have consequences that last a lifetime. If, for example, a child develops a hyperactive fear function, the function is easier triggered later in life, which means that experiences will tend to cause further development of the fear submodule and concomitant anxiety problems.

Whatever mental 'scars' one may have, the situation is never hopeless. The adult mind is sufficiently malleable to make an effort sensible, but a positive start can save the person for considerable effort later in life. The set point has been compared to the situation regarding weight. We all have an innate tendency to end up somewhere on a scale from skinny to obese, but it is possible to lose (or gain) many kilos by a focused, and preferably educated, effort. If, however, the genes— or early life diet—points in the direction of obesity, the effort to turn the trend is more difficult.

As further support for the idea that innate dispositions can be overturned by environmental factors, it may be pointed to the development of stature. The heritability estimates for height range from 0.6 to 0.9 (Silventoinen et al. 2003), which is considerably higher than the 0.3–0.4 heritability of happiness discussed in Sect. 3.5. Yet, in the Netherlands, for example, the average size has moved from five foot four to more than six feet over the last 150 years, primarily due to improved nutrition (Fogel 2005). One would expect that the average level of happiness can also be elevated if we manage to create the right environment.

In the previous section, I suggested that the average level of happiness in an industrialised society is below what was normal for a Stone Age population living in a favourable environment. Whether this conjecture is correct or not, it should be possible to elevate the present level. The arguably more important element is to create an environment that does not bring about undesirable activity in the negative mood module. That is, an environment without the causal discords.

The difficult question is what are the relevant discords? Or, how can we improve the environment in the direction that it moves the mood modules toward a positive output? I shall briefly discuss the possible environmental factors that may affect the three punishment submodules mentioned above, but first a note on exercise.

It is common knowledge that the size and strength of muscles will improve by training, but also neuronal tissue may expand upon use. The point is easily demonstrated in animals where it is possible to apply experimentally controlled stimuli and subsequently remove the brain for detailed anatomical analyses (Hensch 1999). This principle has also been confirmed in humans; for example, hippocampal grey matter is increased as a consequence of exercising navigational skills (Maguire et al. 2000). It has been documented that a finger exercise aimed at improving piano performance leads to enlargement of the motor areas of the brain representing the fingers; and, interestingly, simply imagining the same exercise without moving the fingers leads to comparable changes (Pascual-Leone et al. 2005).

The brain is reasonably plastic and will adapt and improve by a variety of training regimes (Slagter et al. 2011). It seems reasonable to assume that by exercising a brain module—in the form of activating it regularly—it may not only expand, but also have a greater impact on consciousness.

The above conjecture leads to the next question: What cause the modules concerned with negative feelings to develop and thereby gain unwarranted impact on the mind?

It should be pointed out that activation of nerve circuits is somewhat different from activating a muscle. The strengthening of brain modules due to 'exercise' (or, if one prefers, training or learning), is not necessarily a question of anatomical expansion of tissue. It may, for example, be a matter of increasing the number of synapses, pruning or strengthening them, or even atrophy of certain regions. Depression, for example, is associated with decreased activity (and reduced size) in certain parts of the brain (Panksepp 1998; Savitz et al. 2011). Yet, in the present terminology the low mood module is still activated and strengthened, perhaps as a consequence of reduced activity in circuits designed to turn the module off.

Fear. I have previously suggested a possible explanation for why anxiety has become such a common problem in Western societies (Grinde 2005). Briefly, Stone Age people presumably would stay in close proximity to their children, carrying them around during the daytime and sleeping next to them at night, as tribal people tend to do today (McKenna et al. 1999). In modern societies, infants typically spend much time without a sensation of where the parents are, as exemplified by the sleeping arrangements where the infants are placed in their own cribs and often in separate rooms. If children cry when put to bed, a dominant line of thought has been that it is best to ignore their crying in order to teach them to sleep alone (Reid et al. 1999). Following this advice, the baby will eventually stop crying; however, the situation may, over time, spur excessive development of the fear function. Activation of fear, particularly of the type referred to as separation distress, may also follow as a consequence of other aspects of modern living, such as the use of day-care centres.

Infants rely on parental help to avoid any sort of danger, whether in the form of burglars or wild beasts, thus they are not designed to understand that a locked door implies safety. The key to avoid fear is to have the parents close by—the preferred distance is skin-to-skin. The present way of handling infants typically involves reduced parental proximity, e.g., strollers instead of carrying (Fig. 5.1).

Another relevant mismatch concerns the amount of skin contact that infants receive. In the Palaeolithic age, there would be limited use of clothing, and more handling and carrying against the body (Hewlett 1991). In a comparison between

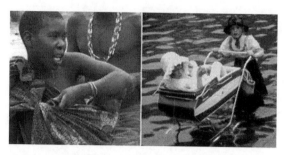

Fig. 5.1 A main element of the present strategy aimed at improving quality of life is to avoid discords that cause excessive activity in punishment submodules. Anxiety-inducing situations are prime candidates; as, for example, the difference between carrying the child skin-to-skin or in a baby stroller. The former is expected to calm the infant. (Photo: B. Grinde)

African tribal people with neighbouring farmers, closer infant care in the tribal group (including more carrying) correlated with less crying and more smiling (Hewlett et al. 1998). Moreover, skin-to-skin contact is known to calm people (Panksepp 1998; Montagu 1978; Anderson and Taylor 2011; Vincent 2011). Thus, a decrease in the dose of either nursing or other forms of touch may contribute to anxiety disorders.

It is well documented that obvious stressful conditions, such as abuse or separation from the mother, can lead to anxiety- and mood-related disorders in both humans and animals—an issue often related to what is referred to as attachment theory (Heim et al. 2000; Bremne and Vermetten 2001; Pryce and Feldon 2003; van der Horst and van 2008). In fact, this form of stress has recently been related to changes in the orbitofrontal cortex, a part of the brain associated with the mood modules (Hanson et al. 2010). However, the prevalence of these disorders in humans appears to be much higher than the prevalence of serious child abuse or neglect. Moreover, most patients do not report such a background. Thus, even in the case of what is presently considered a normal upbringing, there are likely to be practises and cultural traditions that contribute to an increase in anxiety. Milder forms of stress, such as insisting that the infant shall sleep alone at night, may not lead to distinct changes in the brain, but still cause an increased vulnerability to anxiety.

It is important to note that the question is not whether the environments the babies are offered are hazardous. Both day-care centres and modern housing may very well be safer than Palaeolithic campsites. The point is that infants are prone to respond to the absence of parental proximity as a threat, while not responding to more imminent dangers simply because they have evolved to rely on parental effort to escape.

Low mood. In Sect. 4.2, I suggested that the low mood module is activated when the social network is lacking, or when one fails at a task. Thus, the high prevalence of depression may reflect that modern societies are troubled by a suboptimal social environment, as well as by too much pressure on achievements that are difficult to attain. Altering these conditions may reduce excessive exercise of the low mood module.

Possibly the most obvious discord, as well as one of the most common complaints, is simply that of loneliness and lack of belonging. People do not develop positive community relations of the strength and duration evolution has shaped our mind to expect. In the tribal world of the Stone Age, most individuals had life-long connections with a handful of others—whom they depended on for survival. It is difficult to achieve an equally close-knit commune in a modern industrialised country. Frequent encounters with dominant and intimidating individuals—such as teachers and bosses—may lead to further expansion of the low mood module.

The present social structure is likely to amplify conflicts, both at the group level and at the individual level. The 'tragedy of the commons' is the story of how shared pastures get destroyed as a result of overgrazing because farmers are unwilling to limit the number of animals. The story is used as a metaphor for a general lack of collaboration (Hardin 1968). In the Stone Age, collaboration was presumably easier due to the closer ties between the individuals involved. Conflicts did arise, but the present high population density and concomitant decrease in relations between people are likely discords affecting the level of cooperation achieved. As for the individual level, while conflicts in the Stone Age probably tended to find resolution, today they can last a lifetime. You do not depend on your neighbour for survival, neither do you have a life-long commitment with him; consequently, the quarrels that arise are more difficult to settle. Unresolved disputes can have a considerable negative impact on life.

Anxiety and depression are related conditions, as seen in their comorbidity (Kessler et al. 2005); and as the two reflect related submodules of brain punishment, the connection between the two is also reflected in the recent observation that depression may be due to reduced adult neurogenesis in the hippocampus as a consequence of an elevated level of glucocorticoid hormones delivered by the adrenal gland due to fear (see Fig. 4.2) (Snyder et al. 2011).

Pain. Chronic pain affects some 20% of the adult European population (Breivik et al. 2006). The prevalence increases considerably with age. It is therefore difficult to tell whether the problem is a natural consequence of ageing, and that the high prevalence simply reflects the present age profile of the population, or whether discord conditions contribute to the prevalence. It is also often difficult to know whether the pain is functional, for example by helping the individual avoid further damage to the issue in question.

That said, it seems plausible that discords are responsible for part of the problem. Possible discords include unnatural physical activity (either lack of such or chronic strain on certain parts of the body), as well as an overactive inflammatory response. As discussed elsewhere, the latter may reflect discords in the way we interact with microorganisms—an idea sometimes referred to as the 'hygiene hypothesis' (Okada et al. 2010).

It is interesting to note that chronic pain correlates with an increased sensitivity towards pain other than the one reported as chronic (Nielsen et al. 2009). The observation supports the idea that uncalled-for 'exercise' of the pain submodule may contribute. In fact, chronic pain has been associated with a form of learning referred to as long-term potentiation (Zhuo 2007), and with hyperactivity in negative mood-related structures such as the amygdala and anterior cingulate cortex (Porreca and Price 2009).

As I have argued in more detail elsewhere, it seems unlikely that the present prevalence of anxiety, depression and chronic pain reflects a natural condition for the human species (Grinde 2009). A common denominator of the causes suggested above is that they reflect ways of living in industrialised societies that differ from the way of life in the Stone Age. Consequently, the problems may be viewed as stemming from environmental conditions that are at discord with how the human species is genetically adapted to live. Research aimed at evaluating the relative role, if any, of the putative discords I have listed would be timely; as exemplified by the research aimed at investigating the causal role of discord diet and physical activity in mood disorders mentioned in Sect. 4.2.

5.2 Exercising the Brain

The present model of the brain implies that a suitable upbringing—that is, a non-discord environment—should leave an 'unscarred' brain and thus a (natural) positive level of happiness due to the notion of default contentment. Preventive measures (i.e., avoiding discords such as those suggested in the previous section) are obviously to be preferred compared to therapeutic options—particularly in the case of mental disorders for which treatment is generally difficult. Thus adjusting the environment should be the first priority, but this strategy alone is not expected to yield optimal life quality—for two reasons:

1. It seems unlikely that we can retain the advantages of an industrialised society without accepting some discords.
2. It should be possible to elevate the level of happiness beyond the natural set point of the individual.

Most likely no Stone Age person was ever able to run a 100 metres in less than 10 s, or a marathon in just about 2 h. With the advent of ever more efficient training regimes, people keep breaking the world records in sport. Likewise, if we are able to design optimal training methods for the mind, it should be possible to gain a level of happiness beyond any previous society, and above what the innate disposition would suggest. This chapter will discuss the possible options.

The brain is a particularly malleable organ, thus with the right effort, it is theoretically possible to alleviate most psychological problems. Unfortunately, it is not easy, which is why mental disorders are so common.

The arguably most successful form of treatment is cognitive therapy, which has been shown to improve conditions related to anxiety and depression. Yet, few patients are completely healed; and life-long treatment is common.

In Sect. 4.2 I used the example of myopia. Although there are clues as to what is causing its high prevalence in Western societies, there has not been much interest in changing the suggested discords. Then again, compared to mental problems, myopia is easy to diagnose, and easy to mend. Consequently, finding (and improving) the discord conditions responsible for a suboptimal mind is much more important. Unfortunately, both in the case of myopia, and as regards mental problems, finding the cause is difficult; which means that society must be prepared for having a considerable fraction of the population troubled by mental disorders and concomitant unhappiness.

The pertinent question is then whether there are alleviating measures that does not require high costs for the health authorities. Certain forms of brain exercise may offer an opportunity.

The subconscious delivers information to the conscious brain on a 'need to know basis'. Similarly, delegation of control over mental and bodily functions is limited to what was useful during the evolution of our species; i.e., the brain is not designed to render full command to the whims of consciousness. If, for example, the sight of an elevator activates claustrophobic fear, the sufferer is typically unable to turn it off. It is possible to impact on the mood modules in the direction of subduing the anxiety; but it requires, in general, an effort over a long period.

A key point is that the brain presumably not only has structures designed to turn *on* positive and negative feelings, but also to turn them *off*. The obvious purpose of the latter is to disengage pains and pleasures when these are no longer appropriate. Hedonic pleasures, for example, will eventually become less pleasurable when gorged on, as the instigating delight signal is no longer relevant for the genes. When the stomach is full, you should stop eating. Similarly, pain and fear should be turned off when no longer useful; for example, when they are not needed to prevent further inflictions, or when the 'snake' turned out to be a stick. Otherwise the negative mood will hamper activity required for sustenance.

The brain structures, or modules, designed to turn off feelings may also be exercised and strengthened. Cognitive therapy is, in the present terminology, one way of boosting the deactivation neural circuits. It has proven particularly successful in treating certain forms of anxiety. Exposure is often a key element of this therapy, as it allows for exercise of the 'disengage module'. For example, the claustrophobic patient is asked to first simply stand outside an elevator until he can tackle that situation without anxiety; for later to move inside while focusing on stopping the fear. The concept of 'fear extinction' presumably reflects exercise of the turn-off-fear-module, and glucocorticoids may enhance the process (de Quervain et al. 2011). Presumably the same principle applies to a mountain climber who learns to control the fear of heights.

The therapy, or exercise, meant to alleviate the situation could work either by blocking (or unlearning) the stimuli from instigating fear, or by strengthening the capacity to turn the fear signal off at an early stage. Research suggests, however, that the latter type of process is the more important (Hofmann 2008).

The high prevalence of non-functional pain, anxiety and depression suggests that the system of activation and deactivation does not always function according

Fig. 5.2 Meditation may
offer the equivalent of an
exercise machine in a fitness
centre when it comes to
training the mind. (Photo:
B. Grinde)

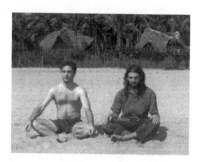

to the intention. Apparently, it is more likely that the various submodules turning on punishment have elevated activity, compared to those meant to turn it off. The cause of this situation may be related to discords. In the case of fear, for example, dangerous situations were originally more likely to be an event with a clear 'endpoint'. The attack of a predator would soon be over, while we face traffic and strangers, angry neighbours, bills and exams, on a more continuous basis. In other words, today more anxiety may stem from situations that linger and have no distinct conclusion. The deactivation circuitry is consequently not sufficiently engaged. That is to say, the cause of anxiety may be brought down to a misbalance between the modules activating fear and those deactivating it.

Human ingenuity allows us to try to amend the problem, as exemplified by cognitive therapy. Fortunately, the brain is not necessarily that difficult to sway. The point is illustrated by the power of the placebo effect in the treatment of mental disorders. Yet, amending a scarred brain requires an effort—the person needs to know how to deal with the problem, and to set aside time.

Besides cognitive therapy, a range of strategies are aimed at improving mental health and happiness. The strategies include older techniques, such as autogenic training, hypnotherapy, yoga and meditation; as well as various cognitive approaches based on the advance of positive psychology, such as self-determination (Niemiec et al. 2009), optimism (Seligman and Csikszentmihalyi 2000; Lyubomirsky et al. 2011) and practising positive emotions (Cohn and Fredrickson 2010). There is no space here to adequately review the field of positive psychology, but I shall take a closer look at meditation because it serves to illustrate the potential for exercising the mind. Meditative techniques, including mindfulness, are particularly interesting in relation to the present model (Fig. 5.2).

As reviewed by McGee (2008), there is reasonable evidence suggesting that meditation has a potential for improving mental health. While most types of mental training, such as learning to play the piano or memorising cards, tend to be restricted to a narrow range of tasks, meditation may work as a more general exercise—directed, for example, at improving attention (Slagter et al. 2011; Tang and Posner 2009). Besides improved attention, a main target may be to reduce stress by working on the capacity to 'relax the mind'. Those who meditate regularly have changes in brain activity associated with improved mental health

(Brewer et al. 2011), as well as lower levels of the stress hormone cortisol, and changes in the amygdala suggestive of a reduced fear response (Holzel et al. 2010).

Meditation seems to offer a 'gateway to the mind' for implementing changes that are not easily achieved by traditional learning. It may be a question of turning off or tuning down, cognitive activity; and consequently leaving the mind more open for focused exercise of a particular module; or perhaps enhance brain plasticity (Xiong and Doraiswamy 2009). Although most practitioners focus on the calming, 'turning off thoughts' part—which may primarily work on stress and anxiety—some use mediation to improve specific elements of the mind. Tibetan Buddhists, for example, typically focus their meditation on love and compassion. As pointed out in Sect. 2.3, empathy and social connections induce powerful brain rewards (Grinde 2009).

It is also possible to focus more directly on the reward modules; as when trying to induce an 'I-feel-good' attitude during the meditation. Both this exercise and compassion meditation is expected to improve the mood tonus (or set point of happiness). Practitioners of the Tibetan Buddhist tradition (or the related mindfulness technique) have been investigated to some detail in this respect, using various neurobiological methods such as brain scans. It has been claimed that their practise is capable of installing in the brain a sufficiently strong reward module to allow for a positive sentiment regardless of the external situation (Ricard 2007). The mood elevating effects of meditation are substantiated by measuring changes in brain activity, or morphology, associated with positive feelings (Lutz et al. 2004, 2008; Wallace 2007; Holzel et al. 2011; Salomons and Kucyi 2011).

According to the present model, the main challenge as to improving happiness is to find a way to exercise the salient brain modules. Present forms of meditation are generally based on religious (or other non-scientific) traditions. The techniques have evolved by trial and error, in the form of the personal experiences of various sages. By merging present knowledge of the brain, and of what happiness is about, it may be possible to improve these techniques.

For example, traditional meditation has typically been concerned with finding peace, feeling calm or being in touch with spiritual entities. The person meditates on a meaningless sound (a mantra) or perhaps on a bodily function such as breathing. The evidence suggests that the effort may yield a more relaxed mind, which is a central point in bringing forth the default state of contentment; but it is also possible to direct the meditation more specifically at the mental issues facing the person. That is, to find an exercise catering to the particular submodules that ought to be strengthened.

There are three key issues when it comes to devising an appropriate mental exercise:

1. To pinpoint the module that requires training.
2. To find a way to activate this module.
3. To put the mind in a state where it is more likely to 'absorb' the exercise.

The first is a question of understanding what is troubling the mind. If the problem is related to anxiety, one should try to identify the specific cause (e.g., spiders or social relations), if any; similarly, if the problem is related to low mood, the key may be loneliness or lack of success.

The second issue concerns how to best activate the desired submodule. In the case of anxiety and depression, it is primarily a question of activating the 'turn off' module.

In the Tibetan Buddhist tradition the practitioner meditates on compassion by thinking of someone with empathy and trying to purify this state of the mind. One alternative would be to induce an attitude described as 'let-go-of-worries' in order to turn off anxiety; or simply get into a 'feel-good-state' and try to retain and focus on this sensation. The Bobby McFerrin song 'Don't worry—be happy' may be suitable for many people, whether one prefers to sing it or use the title as a mantra.

The exercise presumably depends on activating the relevant module of the brain—in the case of empathy, to really feel the compassion. This is often difficult, and a relevant, somewhat indirect, strategy is to formulate short sentences such as the one suggested above, and repeat them as a mantra. The text itself is assumed to have an impact, by (subconsciously) stimulating the corresponding part of the mind. Of course, one may preferably at the same time try to get into a corresponding state. Conjuring relevant images in the mind, for example in the form of the person your compassion is directed at, may help the process. The sentences and images presumably offer an 'indirect' route to the desired brain submodules.

The more common use of mantras is more in the line of offering the conscious something to 'hold on to'—a trick that makes it easier to avoid having thoughts interrupt the process, and thereby keep the mind empty or 'floating'. Meditating on a sentence, an attitude or a feeling is a form of focused attention meditation, and is practised in certain traditions (Lutz et al. 2008). The method is related to self-hypnosis (Hammond 2010).

The third point is to enter a state where the mind is particularly malleable. Apparently the classical form of meditation, which implies 'freeing the mind for thoughts and worries' is particularly suitable. Those who do meditate know when they enter a 'meditative' state, and can induce that more or less efficiently at will. The idea that the mind should be as 'empty' as possible may be a clue to why this is a suitable state for brain exercise. If other activity is stopped, it may be possible to direct more attention to the module one tries to work out.

Although most people will benefit from counselling in order to get started with meditation, further practise can be performed without qualified assistance. Once the technique is established, it is possible to use it in various settings, such as while walking or riding a bus. Sitting in a meditative position in a quiet room should, however, yield a better exercise. As the counselling does not need to be one-to-one, meditation is an inexpensive form of treatment.

Neither cognitive therapy, nor meditation or any of the other types of exercise mentioned, may cure all problems; but it seems fair to expect that most people may benefit by an informed effort. I believe that thinking in terms of 'exercising the brain' is useful in this endeavour. It does suggest what features of the process are more likely to yield success.

5.3 Is it Best to be Rational?

The *Age of Reason*, or Age of Rationalism, was a philosophical tradition starting in the seventeenth century. Modern science, and the present sentiment of Western culture, owes a lot to this tradition. We learn in school to be as rational as possible, and base our decisions on empirical evidence and a scientific world view. The question is whether this necessarily is the optimal strategy if the purpose, as I argued in Chap. 1, is to maximise happiness?

Religion is an interesting case that helps outline the issue (Fig. 5.3). Belief in supernatural powers is considered a defining feature of spirituality. Although religious people can be highly rational when dealing with most issues, they typically have at least one belief that non-religious people (or people of other creeds) are likely to consider superstitious or unscientific. So at that point, if nowhere else, they may be considered irrational.

Then again, religiousness tends to correlate with happiness and health (Chida et al. 2009; Grinde 2005; Diener et al. 2011; Cooper et al. 2011; Abdel-Khalek 2010). It seems likely that this effect is at least partly related to the irrational aspects of faith. For example, belief in an afterlife, or in a protective God, may reduce anxiety; having God as a friend and companion may reduce loneliness and so on. The non-religious will typically argue in disfavour of such practises; but the traditions do seem to cater to the human psyche in a positive way. The disparity raises the following question: Is it irrational to be rational at all times?

Or, to pose the question in a less provocative way: Given that happiness (in the present definition) is what we ought to strive for, should we sometimes let (irrational) thoughts and feelings guide us, rather than taking the most rational stance? Realism may not always be best for your health, optimists have better recovery from operations and live longer (Aspinwall and Tedeschi 2010); and, as pointed out in the previous section, self-hypnotism can improve well-being.

The behaviourism traditions in psychology claim (at its most extreme) that humans are born as blank slates that are subsequently written on (or shaped) by parents and teachers. If this was the case, then happiness could be achieved by means of traditional education. The biologist perspective, however, points out that we are born with innate tendencies to feelings that are not easily overwritten by the environment. In this view, irrational faith may cater better to the human psyche than rational teaching. That is, religion may hit innate tendencies in the brain in ways that are beyond the means of a standard school—to the effect of having a happier population.

Note that religion cannot easily be utilised by a rational stance; for example in the form of deciding that 'I from now on believe in heaven because it is good for me'. To derive advantage from faith, one ought to entertain it wholeheartedly—considering it a rational choice is unlikely to work.

The scientific tradition tends to claim that religion is a way of fooling people in the direction of superstition, inappropriate belief and subsequent adverse behaviour. The argument may be relevant, but if having faith in the supernatural makes

Fig. 5.3 Research suggests
that being religious improves
health and quality of life, but
at the same time many people
consider it irrational. If so,
what is to be preferred?
(Photo: B. Grinde)

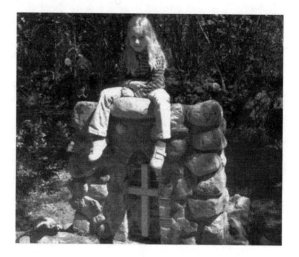

you happier and healthier, the atheists should have second thoughts about trying to obliterate all creeds. As I have argued in more depth elsewhere, it is better to try to mould religion into a more optimal entity for the sake of improving quality of life (Grinde 2005, 2011).

Most of the critiques raised against faith are directed at the two dominant creeds today, Christianity and Islam. It has been estimated that mankind has devised some 100,000 different creeds (Wallace 1966), presumably most of the present criticism is irrelevant in a majority of these cases. Some credos presumably serve the purpose (of improving the conditions for mankind) better than others, but it is also possible to modify suboptimal doctrines. Although Christianity and Islam tend to be conservative as cultural entities, they are not immune to change; thus it should be possible to derive at better interpretations and practises related to the Holy Scriptures.

Another topic serves to further illustrate the dilemma of whether rationality is to be preferred. One may ask whether people ought to fall in love, as opposed to finding a wife or husband based on a scientific strategy of optimal partner choice.

As I have discussed elsewhere, the 'falling in love' module appears to be a unique human adaptation designed to promote couple forming with a partner from another tribe (as part of an evolutionary designed out-breading programme) (Grinde 2002). Love is connected with very powerful brain rewards, but at the same time tends to diminish logical thinking in relation to the characteristics of the partner. A more realistic evaluation might lead to better marriages, but would most likely deprive the person of the wonderful feeling of being in love. Moreover, the love component at least starts the relationship on a positive track. Thus the couple is likely to benefit from the rosy-coloured, irrational impression of the partner. If the choice of a rational stance is available, it is not obvious that it would improve the overall score of happiness. Falling in love fits better with the reward modules of the brain.

As already pointed out, the brain is not designed to promote rationality at all times. We have all sorts of innate tendencies that drive our choices and behaviour. In fact, the average citizen is not at all that good at making decisions directed at maximising lifetime happiness (Gilovitch et al. 2002; Hsee and Hastie 2006). The point is illustrated by risk behaviour: We smoke, abuse alcohol and take chances in relation to sexually transmittable diseases. Most people know the dangers; still the subsequent reduction in disability-adjusted life years (DALY) and life quality is substantial. Rather than opting for long-term contentment, we jump at short-term pleasures (Kimball 1993).

Evolution shaped our innate tendencies to fit the demands of survival and procreation in a Stone Age world. Even then people probably had a tendency to grab opportunities as they appeared—to go for immediate gratification. In an industrialised world this has become a major problem. All sorts of gratifications are readily available, but taking advantage of them to the extent our innate tendencies would suggest, is likely to have a high cost in terms of long-term health and contentment.

Other examples of non-optimal tendencies of choice include: We will pay more to eliminate a small risk of illness than to reduce a large one, more to insure ourselves against a scary way of dying than against every way of dying, and we will save all the members of a five person group rather than six members of a ten person group (Gilbert 2011). The notion of optimising benefits would call for different decisions.

In short, we make inappropriate or suboptimal choices because our innate tendencies are not adapted to a modern world.

As an extension of the above discussion on rationality, it is relevant to note how subconscious nerve circuits may impact on the mood modules.

One example concerns a study that asked students to keep a pencil either between the lips or between the teeth while reading cartoons (Strack et al. 1988). Those with the pencil between the teeth subsequently rated the cartoons as more funny. By having the pencil in the teeth, they forced the lips into a smile (without knowing it). Presumably the smile muscles send signals to the brain saying that the mood is good, which is sufficient to have an impact on the actual mood (Fig. 5.4).

Likewise, forcing laughter (Shahidi et al. 2011), or blocking a frown (Lewis and Bowler 2009), appears to be sufficient to boost happiness.

These studies suggest that our emotions are reinforced—perhaps to some extent even driven—by their corresponding (facial) expressions; a point reflected in the writings of Darwin: 'The free expression by outward signs of an emotion intensifies it' (Darwin 1872, p. 366).

The power of the subconscious is further illustrated by experiments showing that a placebo pill can have an effect even if the patient is told that he is receiving a placebo (Kaptchuk et al. 2010). This result suggests that any 'treatment', including a glass of water or a touch on the shoulder, may work if one can tune the brain to believe it might work. One of the authors, Kirsch, recommends visualising the desired improvement, and telling yourself that something is going to get better (Marchant 2011)—in the present terminology it is a question of exercising the relevant brain module.

Fig. 5.4 Putting a pencil between the teeth rather than between the lips forces the mouth to produce a smile. The person does not need to be aware of the smile, yet it can influence the mood modules of the brain. Apparently the smile muscles send feedback to the brain saying 'you are smiling, thus you are happy'. (Photo: B. Grinde)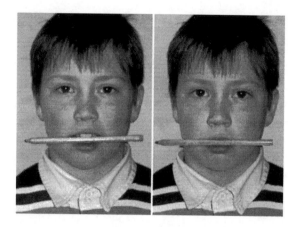

The conscious mind can be used to initiate processes presumably belonging to the subconscious, to the effect that changes occur that are relevant to how we feel. In short, we can modulate the activity of the mood modules.

Although understanding the human mind can lead to improved quality of life, the rational choice may sometimes be to let the subconscious tendencies retain their influence, as when falling in love. In other situations, the winning strategy is to curb innate impulses; for example in connection with overt rage and unhealthy eating habits. It is also possible to impact on the subconscious in order to strengthen modules involved in mood—for example by meditating. In other words, the pursuit of happiness is a considerable challenge.

The problems can be attributed to the following two issues:

1. We are not designed by evolution for the sake of our quality of life.
2. We are not designed to live in an industrialised society.

It is, fortunately, possible to take advantage of how the mind is constructed. By employing human ingenuity, we can improve our score of happiness. For this purpose we need to understand the biology of wellbeing. The present perspective suggests five ways of bending the mind in order to improve mental health and life quality:

1. 'You are what you think'. By positive thinking, and by cultivating (minor) pleasures, the underlying brain circuits are exercised. In fact, positive thinking can have health benefits of a strength comparable to the negative effect of stress and pessimism (Chida and Steptoe 2008).
2. Boost your ego. It helps to have high opinions of oneself. Those who see themselves in a positive light, have lower markers of stress, such as baseline cortisol, and recover faster from stressful situations (Taylor et al. 2003).
3. Find time for specific exercise of problematic or suboptimal modules—particularly those involved in turning off punishment. Meditative techniques can enhance the effect of the exercise. Even short periods should make a difference, perhaps 5 min a couple of times each day where meditative techniques are mixed with specific activation of relevant modules.

4. Build strong social connections. If you fail with humans, try a dog, a cat or a god. Curing loneliness may be as important for health as quitting smoking (Hawkley and Cacioppo 2010). The important point may be not so much the number of friends, but the feeling of having someone who can be called upon when needed, as well as not being surrounded by hostile people.

5. Find a decent religion and engage in it—in order to take advantage of the (imaginary) companionship offered, the (real) social life of the congregation, the sense of belonging, the notion of a protective entity and finding a meaning in life.

The first step to happiness is knowing thyself. If the knowledge is at hand, the second step requires the willpower to act. The question is not so much 'to be or not to be', but rather 'when to be rational, and when not to be'—and 'how to be happy, and how not to be'.

The pertinent issues of this chapter can be summarised as follows:

1. Most bodily functions can be exercised. In the case of brain functions, exercise typically results in a stronger module with more impact on the conscious self.

2. Whether or not the level of happiness was better in the Stone Age than today, it should be possible to improve the score.

3. One ought to avoid discords that cause exercise of the main punishment modules: fear, low mood and pain.

4. Lack of proximity and skin contact between infants and parents are key discords regarding anxiety, a frail social network as well as failure in tasks are relevant discords in connection with depression, and physical activity and altered relations to microbes in relation to pain.

5. The brain contains both on and off switches for the various mood modules. The training should be aimed at turning on positive feelings and off inappropriate negative feelings.

6. Cognitive therapy has proven particularly useful in helping people turn off anxiety. Meditation may work as an 'exercise machine' for the mind and a range of other techniques for positive training are also available.

7. If happiness is the ultimate purpose, rationality is at times irrational. Behavioural options that cater to certain innate tendencies, from religion to falling in love, may yield a better score of happiness compared to a logical stance.

8. The subconscious brain can impact on the mood modules in a variety of ways.

References

Abdel-Khalek, A. M. (2010). Quality of life, subjective well-being, and religiosity in Muslim college students. *Quality of Life Research, 19*, 1133–1143.

Anderson, J. G., & Taylor, A. G. (2011). Effects of healing touch in clinical practice: Asystematic review of randomized clinical trials. *Journal of Holistic Nursing, 29*, 221–228.

Aspinwall, L. G., & Tedeschi, R. G. (2010). The value of positive psychology for health psychology: Progress and pitfalls in examining the relation of positive phenomena to health. *Annals of Behavioral Medicine, 39*, 4–15.

Breivik, H., Collett, B., Ventafridda, V., Cohen, R., & Gallacher, D. (2006). Survey of chronic pain in Europe: Prevalence, impact on daily life, and treatment. *European Journal of Pain, 10,* 287–333.

Bremne, J. D., & Vermetten, E. (2001). Stress and development: Behavioral and biological consequences. *Development and Psychopathology, 13,* 473–489.

Brewer, J. A., Worhunsky, P. D., Gray, J. R., Tang, Y. Y., Weber, J., & Kober, H. (2011). Meditation experience is associated with differences in default mode network activity and connectivity. *Proceedings of the National Academy of Sciences U S A, 108,* 20254–20259.

Chida, Y., & Steptoe, A. (2008). Positive psychological well-being and mortality: A quantitative review of prospective observational studies. *Psychosomatic Medicine, 70,* 741–756.

Chida, Y., Steptoe, A., & Powell, L. H. (2009). Religiosity/spirituality and mortality. A systematic quantitative review. *Psychother Psychosom, 78,* 81–90.

Cohn, M. A., & Fredrickson, B. L. (2010). In search of durable positive psychology interventions: Predictors and consequences of long-term positive behavior change. *Journal of Positive Psychology, 5,* 355–366.

Cooper, C., Bebbington, P., King, M., Jenkins, R., Farrell, M., Brugha, T., et al. (2011). Happiness across age groups: Results from the 2007 National Psychiatric Morbidity Survey. *International Journal of Geriatric Psychiatry, 26,* 608–614.

Darwin, C. (1872). *The expression of emotions in man and animals.* London: John Murray.

de Quervain, D. J., Bentz, D., Michael, T., Bolt, O. C., Wiederhold, B. K., & Margraf, J., et al. (2011). Glucocorticoids enhance extinction-based psychotherapy. *Proceedings of the National Academy of Sciences U S A, 108,* 6621–6625.

Diener. E., Tay, L., & Myers, D.G. (2011). The religion paradox: If religion makes people happy, why are so many dropping out? *Journal of Personality and Social Psychology, 101*(6): 1278–9120

Fogel, R. W. (2005). Changes in the disparities in chronic diseases during the course of the 20th century. *Perspectives in Biology and Medicine, 48,* S150–S165.

Gilbert, D. (2011). Buried by bad decisions. *Nature, 474,* 275–277.

Gilovitch, T., Griffin, D., & Kahneman, D. (2002). *Heuristics and biases: Psychology of intuitive judgement.* Cambridge: Cambridge University Press.

Grinde, B. (2002). *Darwinian happiness - Evolution as a guide for living and understanding human behavior.* Princeton: The Darwin Press.

Grinde, B. (2005a). An approach to the prevention of anxiety-related disorders based on evolutionary medicine. *Preventive Medicine, 40,* 904–909.

Grinde, B. (2005b). Can science promote religion for the benefit of society? How can science help religion toward optimal benefit for society? *Zygon, 40,* 277–288.

Grinde, B. (2009a). Can the concept of discords help us find the causes of mental diseases? *Medical Hypotheses, 73,* 106–109.

Grinde, B. (2009b). An evolutionary perspective on the importance of community relations for quality of life. *ScientificWorldJournal, 9,* 588–605.

Grinde, B. (2011). *God: A scientific update.* Princeton: The Darwin Press.

Hammond, D. C. (2010). Hypnosis in the treatment of anxiety—and stress-related disorders. *Expert Review of Neurotherapeutics, 10,* 263–273.

Hanson, J. L., Chung, M. K., Avants, B. B., Shirtcliff, E. A., Gee, J. C., & Davidson, R. J., et al. (2010). Early stress is associated with alterations in the orbitofrontal cortex: A tensor-based morphometry investigation of brain structure and behavioral risk. *Journal of Neuroscience, 30,* 7466–7472.

Hardin, G. (1968). The Tragedy of the Commons. *Science, 162,* 1243–1248.

Hawkley, L. C., & Cacioppo, J. T. (2010). Loneliness matters: A theoretical and empirical review of consequences and mechanisms. *Annals of Behavioral Medicine, 40,* 218–227.

Heim, C., Newport, D. J., Heit, S., Graham, Y. P., Wilcox, M., & Bonsall, R., et al. (2000). Pituitary-adrenal and autonomic responses to stress in women after sexual and physical abuse in childhood. *JAMA, 284,* 592–597.

Hensch, T. K. (1999). Whisking away space in the brain. *Neuron, 24,* 492–493.

Hewlett, B. S. (1991). Demography and childcare in preindustrial societies. *Journal of Anthropological Research, 47*, 1–37.

Hewlett, B. S., Lamb, M. E., Shannon, D., Leyendecker, B., & Scholmerich, A. (1998). Culture and early infancy among central African foragers and farmers. *Developmental Psychology, 34*, 653–661.

Hofmann, S. G. (2008). Cognitive processes during fear acquisition and extinction in animals and humans:Implications for exposure therapy of anxiety disorders. *Clinical Psychology Review, 28*, 199–210.

Holzel, B. K., Carmody, J., Evans, K. C., Hoge, E. A., Dusek, J. A., & Morgan, L., et al. (2010). Stress reduction correlates with structural changes in the amygdala. *Social Cognitive and Affective Neuroscience, 5*, 11–17.

Holzel, B. K., Carmody, J., Vangel, M., Congleton, C., Yerramsetti, S. M., & Gard, T., et al. (2011). Mindfulness practice leads to increases in regional brain gray matter density. *Psychiatry Research, 191*, 36–43.

Hsee, C. K., & Hastie, R. (2006). Decision and experience: Why don't we choose what makes us happy? *Trends in Cognitive Sciences, 10*, 31–37.

Kaptchuk, T. J., Friedlander, E., Kelley, J. M., Sanchez, M. N., Kokkotou, E.,& Singer, J. P., et al. (2010). Placebos without deception: A randomized controlled trial in irritable bowel syndrome. *PLoS ONE, 5*, e15591.

Kessler, R. C., Chiu, W. T., Demler, O., Merikangas, K. R., & Walters, E. E. (2005). Prevalence, severity, and comorbidity of 12-month DSM-IV disorders in the National Comorbidity Survey Replication. *Archives of General Psychiatry, 62*, 617–627.

Kimball, M. S. (1993). Standard Risk-Aversion. *Econometrica, 61*, 589–611.

Lewis, M. B., & Bowler, P. J. (2009). Botulinum toxin cosmetic therapy correlates with a more positive mood. *Journal of Cosmetic Dermatology, 8*, 24–26.

Lucas, R. (2008). Personality and subjective well-being. In M. Eid & R. Larsen (Eds.), *The science of subjective well-being* (pp. 171–194). New York: Guilford Press.

Lutz, A., Brefczynski-Lewis, J., Johnstone, T., & Davidson, R. J. (2008a). Regulation of the neural circuitry of emotion by compassion meditation: Effects of meditative expertise. *PLoS ONE, 3*, e1897.

Lutz, A., Greischar, L. L., Rawlings, N. B., Ricard, M., & Davidson, R. J. (2004). Long-term meditators self-induce high-amplitude gamma synchrony during mental practice. *Proceedings of the National Academy of Sciences U S A, 101*, 16369–16373.

Lutz, A., Slagter, H. A., Dunne, J. D., & Davidson, R. J. (2008b). Attention regulation and monitoring in meditation. *Trends in Cognitive Sciences, 12*, 163–169.

Lykken, D. (2000). *Happiness: The nature and nurture of joy and contentment*. New York: St. Martin's Griffin.

Lyubomirsky, S., Dickerhoof, R., Boehm, J. K., & Sheldon, K. M. (2011). Becoming happier takes both a will and a proper way: An experimental longitudinal intervention to boost well-being. *Emotion, 11*, 391–402.

Maguire, E. A., Gadian, D. G., Johnsrude, I. S., Good, C. D., Ashburner, J., & Frackowiak, R. S., et al. (2000). Navigation-related structural change in the hippocampi of taxi drivers. *Proceedings of the National Academy of Sciences U S A, 97*, 4398–4403.

Marchant, J. (2011). Heal thyself. *New Scientist* 33–36

McGee, M. (2008). Meditation and psychiatry. *Psychiatry, 5*, 28–41.

McKenna, J., Mosko, S., & Richard, C. (1999). Breast feeding and mother-infant cosleeping in relation to SIDS prevention. In W. Trevathan, E. Smith, & J. McKenna (Eds.), *Evolutionary medicine* (pp. 53–74). Oxford: Oxford University Press.

Montagu, A. (1978). *Touching: The human significance of the skin*. New York: Harper & Row.

Nielsen, C. S., Staud, R., & Price, D. D. (2009). Individual differences in pain sensitivity: Measurement, causation, and consequences. *Journal of Pain, 10*, 231–237.

Niemiec, C. P., Ryan, R. M., & Deci, E. L. (2009). The path taken: Consequences of attaining intrinsic and extrinsic aspirations in post-college life. *Journal of Research in Personality, 73*, 291–306.

Okada, H., Kuhn, C., Feillet, H., & Bach, J. F. (2010). The 'hygiene hypothesis' for autoimmune and allergic diseases: An update. *Clinical and Experimental Immunology, 160*, 1–9.

Panksepp, J. (1998). *Affective neruoscience*. New York: Oxford University Press.

Pascual-Leone, A., Amedi, A., Fregni, F., & Merabet, L. B. (2005). The plastic human brain cortex. *Annual Review of Neuroscience, 28*, 377–401.

Porreca, F., & Price, T. (2009). When pain lingers. *Scientific American MIND, 20*(5), 34–41

Pryce, C. R., & Feldon, J. (2003). Long-term neurobehavioural impact of the postnatal environment in rats: Manipulations, effects and mediating mechanisms. *Neuroscience and Biobehavioral Reviews, 27*, 57–71.

Reid, M. J., Walter, A. L., & O'Leary, S. G. (1999). Treatment of young children's bedtime refusal and nighttime wakings: A comparison of "standard" and graduated ignoring procedures. *Journal of Abnormal Child Psychology, 27*, 5–16.

Ricard, M. (2007). *Happiness: A guide to developing life's most important skill*. Boston: Atlantic Books.

Salomons, T. V., & Kucyi, A. (2011). Does meditation reduce pain through a unique neural mechanism? *Journal of Neuroscience, 31*, 12705–12707.

Savitz, J. B., Nugent, A. C., Bogers, W., Roiser, J. P., Bain, E. E., & Neumeister, A., et al. (2011). Habenula volume in bipolar disorder and major depressive disorder: A high-resolution magnetic resonance imaging study. *Biological Psychiatry, 69*, 336–343.

Seligman, M. E., & Csikszentmihalyi, M. (2000). Positive psychology. An introduction. *American Psychologist, 55*, 5–14.

Shahidi, M., Mojtahed, A., Modabbernia, A., Mojtahed, M., Shafiabady, A., & Delavar, A., et al. (2011). Laughter yoga versus group exercise program in elderly depressed women: A randomized controlled trial. *International Journal of Geriatric Psychiatry, 26*, 322–327.

Silventoinen, K., Sammalisto, S., Perola, M., Boomsma, D. I., Cornes, B. K., & Davis, C., et al. (2003). Heritability of adult body height: A comparative study of twin cohorts in eight countries. *Twin Research, 6*, 399–408.

Slagter, H. A., Davidson, R. J., & Lutz, A. (2011). Mental training as a tool in the neuroscientific study of brain and cognitive plasticity. *Frontiers in Human Neuroscience, 5*, 17.

Snyder, J. S., Soumier, A., Brewer, M., Pickel, J., & Cameron, H. A. (2011). Adult hippocampal neurogenesis buffers stress responses and depressive behaviour. *Nature, 476*, 458–461.

Strack, F., Martin, L. L., & Stepper, S. (1988). Inhibiting and facilitating conditions of the human smile: A nonobtrusive test of the facial feedback hypothesis. *Journal of Personality and Social Psychology, 54*, 768–777.

Tang, Y. Y., & Posner, M. I. (2009). Attention training and attention state training. *Trends in Cognitive Sciences, 13*, 222–227.

Taylor, S. E., Lerner, J. S., Sherman, D. K., Sage, R. M., & McDowell, N. K. (2003). Are self-enhancing cognitions associated with healthy or unhealthy biological profiles? *Journal of Personality and Social Psychology, 85*, 605–615.

van der Horst, F. C., & van der Veer, R. (2008). Loneliness in infancy: Harry Harlow, John Bowlby and issues of separation. *Integrative Psychological & Behavioral Science, 42*, 325–335.

Vincent, S. (2011). Skin-to-skin contact. Part one: Just an hour of your time. *Practising Midwife, 14*, 40–41.

Wallace, A. (1966). *Religion: An anthropological view*. New York: Random House.

Wallace, A. (2007). *Contemplative science: Where Buddhism and neuroscience converge*. New York: Columbia University Press.

Xiong, G. L., & Doraiswamy, P. M. (2009). Does meditation enhance cognition and brain plasticity? *Annals of the New York Academy of Sciences, 1172*, 63–69.

Zhuo, M. (2007). A synaptic model for pain: Long-term potentiation in the anterior cingulate cortex. *Molecules and Cells, 23*, 259–271.

Chapter 6
The Politics of Happiness

Abstract In agreement with Greek philosophers, happiness can be understood as what society and individuals ought to strive toward. Bhutan was the first country to take the idea seriously, by adopting a policy striving to maximise gross national happiness rather than gross national product. Recently other countries, including France and England, seem to be following suit. It is difficult to find happiness with money, while social connections are a key factor.

Keywords Contextualism · Individualism · Life quality indexes · Happy planet index · Gross national happiness · Bhutan · Wealth

In line with the Greek philosophers, I have defined happiness as what both society and the individual ought to strive toward. It implies that happiness is the ultimate aim of politics. Society should try to establish conditions conducive to a high quality of life—including health care, infrastructure, meaningful work and sufficient economic means—but preferably keep in mind that these targets are no more than proxies for what really matters. While helping the individual in his or her pursuit of happiness, society should also create a setting (including laws and their accompanying punishment) that directs behaviour towards a common good.

The irrationality of the average person, as discussed in the previous chapter, is an important issue. It is debatable to what extent governments should devise policies aimed at making people take better decisions (Thaler and Sunstein 2008; Trout 2009). The question applies to the more traditional fields of intervention, such as in connection with nutrition, smoking and drinking; and to the somewhat broader scope of avoiding discords. In recent discussions, the view that people fare best when the environment, or context, they live in is constrained by authorities have been referred to as *contextualism*, while *individualism* suggests that people should be allowed to decide for themselves (Haybron 2008). The present model suggests that the ideal is to weigh the negative effects of restricting freedom, against the positive effects of behaviour more conductive to well-being, in order to derive at a compromise that yields optimal average happiness.

B. Grinde, *The Biology of Happiness*, SpringerBriefs in Well-Being and Quality of Life Research, DOI: 10.1007/978-94-007-4393-9_6, © The Author(s) 2012

In order to define the best strategy, the issue of happiness ought to be approached by the full force of modern science. This book is meant to be a step in this direction by creating a model that bridges various scientific approaches. Moreover, I have tried to formulate some general advice as to improving mental health and quality of life.

My own country, Norway, along with the other Scandinavian countries, typically ends up near the top of the lists that rate either subjective well-being or life quality in the world (see, for example, Human Development Index, Human Resources Index and Legatum Prosperity Index—data are available on the Internet). The ratings may be relevant, but in my mind they do not imply that Norway is an ideal society. The country is no exception to the mental disorder statistics discussed in Chap. 4. It is difficult to reconcile a high prevalence of diseases such as anxiety and depression with an optimal level of happiness.

According to WHO statistics, the prevalence of certain mental problems may indeed be higher in Western countries compared to less industrialised societies, but the comparison is technically very difficult (Kessler and Ustun 2008; WHO 2008). The main point is that by exploiting current knowledge, it should be possible to further improve the situation in both developed and developing countries. Measures responding to the problem of discords discussed in Sect 5.1 would be one relevant approach.

It is not obvious that governments are any better than individuals at making rational decisions. The aim of most industrialised societies seems to be more in the direction of increasing gross national product (GNP); that is, to create an environment catering to economic, rather than human, growth. The famous economist John Stuart Mill wrote in his book *Principles of Political Economy* that when a country has reached a reasonable economic level, it is time to stabilise the economy and rather focus on quality of life. The book was published in 1848. His ideas seem to be forgotten by most head of states—recently, however, some have voiced similar thoughts.

In 1972, the fourth king of Bhutan proclaimed that in his country they would not strive towards optimising GNP, but rather to improve gross national happiness (GNH) (Fig. 6.1). The country eventually set up an institute for the purpose of implementing this policy, the Centre for Bhutan Studies, which specifies factors of relevance for GNH and device tools for measuring progress.

The king of Bhutan was not taken seriously at the time, but in 2008, the French Prime Minister Nicholas Sarkozy asked the Nobel Prize winning economist Joseph Stiglitz to evaluate other options than GNP for directing the ambitions of his country. Stiglitz's report concluded with pretty much the same ideas as suggested by the King (Stiglitz et al. 2009). Since then the notion that a country should consider quality of life, rather than simply money, has become increasingly accepted (Seaford 2011).

In further support of the foresightful proclamation of the King, scientists find only a weak correlation between happiness and riches; at least when distinguishing emotional aspects of well-being from 'life evaluation'—which is to say, how successful people consider themselves to be (Kahneman and Deaton 2010;

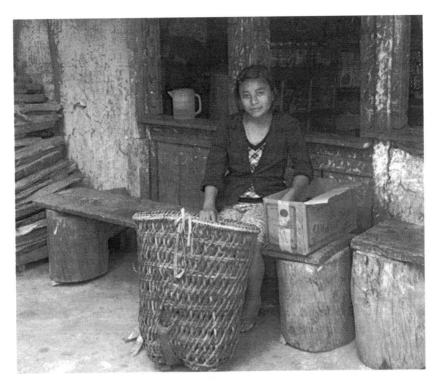

Fig. 6.1 Bhutan—the land of Gross National Happiness. The government says happiness is what they should strive toward. The country is doing quite well, so the initiative seems to carry an impact, although business may be as usual for most people, including this young shopkeeper. (Photo: B. Grinde)

Diener et al. 2010). In a way, money can buy a high personal estimate of success, but not emotional happiness. In poor countries, money does correlate with declared well-being (up to a certain income), but in a country such as the United States even the very rich are only slightly happier than the average person.

Whereas money has only a minor effect on emotional well-being, happiness has been suggested to breed prosperity (Bok 2010); which suggests another reason for promoting well-being rather than wealth. Moreover, following the recommendation of the former king of Bhutan and giving priority to GNH rather than GNP, should help save the Earth for future generations.

On the other hand, one may argue that a sound economy is important to create the means to be happy. Although the basic requirement for life does not require a high income, it is extremely difficult in the present world to operate a society without considering employment and industrial output. A country that does not care about GNP will easily drift onto a very dubious path, where lack of productivity leads to unemployment and social unrest. World dominance goes to the rich and strong states; and the absence of riches (and concomitant luxury) in a setting where most people have money, is likely to cause dissatisfaction. Furthermore, the economic ambitions of individuals are driving the progress in technology and medicine; which in the long run can have considerable impact on life quality. The potential of modern medicine to increase both quantity (years) and quality of life may not be easily visible in studies focusing on subjective well-being, but it does matter if the progress towards further improvements in health services should stop—or the present service decline.

Some societies support high levels of happiness with modest material holdings, for example, Maasai herders, Inughuit hunter-gatherers, and Amish communities (Biswas-Diener et al. 2005; Inglehart et al. 2008; Graham 2009). These societies, however, share one of the following two characteristics:

1. Limited contact with the riches of the Western world, which implies less pressure to 'possess what everybody else possesses'.
2. A strong and permeating ideology that excludes industrial products and purchasing power as something to be pursued.

It seems difficult to introduce these constraints to the rest of the world. It should, however, be possible to slowly shift the sentiment towards thinking more in terms of mental issues rather than economic growth. The priorities and policies suggested by the Centre for Bhutan Studies, the Stiglitz report and The Happy Planet Index from New Economics Foundation (Abdallah et al. 2009) should point in the right direction.

References

Abdallah, S., Thompson, S., Michaelson, J., Marks, N., & Steuer, N. (2009). *The happy planet index 2.0*. London: New Economic Foundation.

Biswas-Diener, R., Vittersø, J., & Diener, E. (2005). Most people are pretty happy, but there is cultural variation: The Inughuit, the Amish, and the Maasai. *Journal of Happiness Studies, 6*, 205–226.

Bok, D. (2010). *The politics of happiness: What government can learn from the new research on well-being*. Princeton: Princeton University Press.

Diener, E., Ng, W., Harter, J., & Arora, R. (2010). Wealth and happiness across the world: Material prosperity predicts life evaluation, whereas psychosocial prosperity predicts positive feeling. *Journal of Personality and Social Psychology, 99*, 52–61.

Graham, C. (2009). *Happiness around the world: The paradox of happy peasants and miserable millionaires*. Oxford: Oxford University Press.

Haybron, D. M. (2008). *The pursuit of unhappiness: The elusive psychology of well-being*. Oxford: Oxford University Press.

Inglehart, R., Foa, R., Peterson, C., & Welzel, C. (2008). Development, freedom, and rising happiness a global perspective (1981–2007). *Perspectives on Psychological Science, 3*, 264–285.

Kahneman, D., & Deaton, A. (2010). High income improves evaluation of life but not emotional well-being. *Proceedings of the National Academy of Sciences U S A, 107*, 16489–16493.

Kessler, R., & Ustun, T. (2008). *The WHO world mental health surveys*. Cambridge: Cambridge University Press.

Seaford, C. (2011). Policy: Time to legislate for the good life. *Nature, 477,* 532–533.

Stiglitz, J., Sen, A., & Fitoussi, J. P. (2009). Report by the commission on the measurement of economic performance and social progress. Paris: CMEPSP.

Thaler, R., & Sunstein, C. (2008). *Nudge: Improving deicsions about health, wealth, and happiness.* New Haven: Yale University Press.

Trout, J. (2009). *The empathy gap: Building bridges to the good life and good society.* New York: Viking Press.

WHO (2008). *The global burden of disese: 2004 update.* Geneva: WHO Press.

Chapter 7
Concluding Remarks

Abstract It should be possible to raise the level of happiness beyond the present level, and beyond what might be expected to be the typical state based on our genetic inheritance. Evolution designs for survival and procreation, but we can take advantage of features evolution has added to our brain, and opt for happiness instead. The key elements in this pursuit are: one, to create an environment that caters to the human psyche by avoiding discords; two, to make sure there is sufficient incentive for production and invention in order to supply people with the necessities of life, and with state-of-the-art medical treatment; and three, to teach people to exercise their brain for the purpose of elevating the net output of the mood modules.

Keywords Reward modules · Punishment · Cognitive therapy · Mental health · Money · Human zoo · Aboriginals · Tribal people · Ecovillage · Intentional company

I have argued in favour of having a single term that encompasses all sorts of positive feelings, from sensual experiences, sexual satisfaction, the joy of achievement and to the experience of empathy. The word chosen here is 'happiness', but it is the principle, and not the actual choice of terminology, that is important. This rationale is based partly on evidence (as detailed in the text) suggesting shared evolutionary history and shared neurobiology for the various types of positive affects, partly on the advantages of having a word that covers human aspirations.

I realise that some people object to the idea of including all mood-related brain activity in a single term. Even those who do consent may dislike the choice of word—rather than happiness I might have opted for the more cumbersome 'positive output from the mood modules'.

I believe most objections are of a semantic nature, and as such primarily a question of how appropriate the semantic choice is. That, however, depends partly on how the brain is organised and partly on the perspective taken. The joy of finding a meaning in life obviously feels quite different from the pleasure of eating a cake. If one wishes to

B. Grinde, *The Biology of Happiness*, SpringerBriefs in Well-Being and Quality of Life Research, DOI: 10.1007/978-94-007-4393-9_7, © The Author(s) 2012

stress dissimilarity, it seems rational to choose separate descriptive terms; while if one wishes to point out shared aspects, i.e. the notion that they all converge on key brain circuitry designed to generate rewards, a common term seems appropriate.

Although I do advocate the present meaning of the term happiness, I should add that it is practical to distinguish between the various categories. Concepts such as hedonic and eudaemonic may be used for one type of categorisation.

It is important to try to describe what ought to be the primary focus of human desire and ambitions. Economic measures may serve as a proxy, or as a means, to improve quality of life; but as argued in this book, the actual target should concern what goes on in people's minds. Optimising the average lifetime happiness of the population seems to be a rational ambition.

In short, I claim that we should strive to enhance the positive output from the mood modules as integrated over a lifetime. I realise that some people may claim that particular aspects of life—such as achievements, family, obeying God, how life is recalled at the end—is more important than happiness (even when accepting that all this factors will be part of the happiness score), or that solely eudaemonic elements should count.

Unfortunately, a theoretical model for happiness does not imply a method for quantifying this quality. The brain is too complicated, and not sufficiently understood, for any neurobiological measure to help much. Moreover, the mood modules are easily and unpredictably swayed in either direction, and thus difficult to gauge or anticipate. Consequently, questionnaires of the type used for subjective well-being still stands as our best shot at appraising the condition. As exemplified by the discussion of fear and grief, I have pointed out that a situation can easily change between a positive or negative affect value. The power of the human cognitive input implies that affect is expected to depend on how a condition is conceived, and how one is coping. It is consequently difficult to indicate the level of happiness based on the kind of emotions felt or the situations experienced.

A flower does not feel joy or pain. In the absence of a nervous system an organism is incapable of experiencing anything. What allows humans to enjoy life is the dichotomy of what is good and bad for the genes, in conjunction with the evolutionary construct of, respectively, positive and negative feelings (rewards and punishment) designed to deal with the two types of situations

Once evolution established emotions as an upgraded version of behavioural control, the mood modules became an integral part of the brain. Presumably, they deliver a constant basal activity, not necessarily recognised as either pleasure or pain, but they can also send the mood up or down. It all depends on external opportunities and dangers, internal homeostasis and cognitive deliberations.

The present model is based on the notion that all forms of pleasure and pain are elaborations of ancient functions of the nervous system designed to deal with, respectively, attraction and avoidance. The practical value of this model rests with the question of whether it can help improve quality of life. The key element here is the viewpoint that it matters how the brain is moulded by experience; i.e. what sort of 'exercise' it receives. Three principles are relevant when it comes to boosting happiness—two of them suggest training regimes, the third is a question of avoidance:

1. Exercise the reward modules, which is primarily a question of activating them. Meditative techniques may help, but any sort of positive feelings—including those evoked by music and aesthetics—imply relevant training.
2. Exercise the modules responsible for turning off punishment. Possible regimes include cognitive therapy and focused meditation.
3. Avoid exercising the punishment module by avoiding relevant discords.

Other mammals most likely have more or less the same repertoire of feeling that we find in humans, including the capacity for a wide range of pleasures and pain (Panksepp 1998). The positive and negative mood values may be stronger in humans; but the more important difference is that humans have the competence to understand, and to use that insight to make the most of the situation.

If the basal needs are cared for, and the conditions are not otherwise adverse, it is presumably in human nature to be good humoured and content. In other words, the normal mental state implies an above neutral balance when adding up the activity of positive and negative mood modules. The ensuing joy of life can be observed in children, but unfortunately many adults seem to have lost their natural state of happiness. Adjusting the way of life in order to escape discords and stress should improve the condition, and may be more important for lifetime score of happiness than the exercises suggested in points 1 and 2 above.

In other words, point 3 is where the shoe pinches, because in the absence of punishing activity, the default state of contentment ought to secure a happy life. As the brain is most malleable during infancy, it is particularly relevant to focus on how children are brought up.

The human body has been compared to a car. In both cases any part or function can go awry; but some parts are more likely to create problems, and some defects have more dire consequences. The brain is perhaps the most delicate and susceptible part of the human body, somewhat like the electrical system of a modern car. There is, however, one main difference between humans and cars: The former has a capacity to mend itself. If a light bulb is gone in the car, it is highly unlikely that it should suddenly start working again.

Unwholesome exercise of negative modules is certainly not the sole explanation for mental disorders; there are several possible causes for suboptimal functioning of the brain. Nonetheless, the notion of brain exercise offers a strategy for ameliorating problems that trouble many people. It implies tuning into the brain's innate capacity to recover and improve.

The principles explained above can be illustrated by hypothetical time curves for happiness (Fig. 7.1).

I have suggested that the excessive stimulation of negative submodules is due to discord aspects of living in an industrialised society. People with either a vulnerable disposition, or with a less suitable way of life, consequently end up with a happiness threatening mental problem. I believe preventive measures, based on the notion of discords, should improve the situation; but they cannot (and should not) obliterate negative feelings. The punishment modules are an important part of human nature, the point is to avoid inappropriate activity.

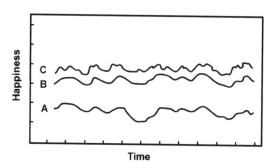

Fig. 7.1 Theoretical time curves for happiness. A: The person scores low on default state of contentment. B and C: The same person going through the same life episodes, but having retained the default contentment. C: With the additional difference of having exercised reward modules and the brain circuits responsible for turning off punishment modules. The curves are solely meant to illustrate principles, thus the scales have no units

The estimated prevalence of anxiety and depression is prone to a more or less arbitrary cut-off as to what is considered abnormal or pathological. However, regardless of where the line is drawn, it seems likely that these punishment modules display considerable non-functional activity in industrialised societies. One would not expect the fear or low mood functions to be designed by evolution in such a way that a substantial fraction of the population suffers from obviously irrational, maladaptive and more or less debilitating anxiety or depression. And even if this assumption should be wrong, the present advice as to avoiding undesirable activity in the negative submodules would be expected to improve quality of life. However, more research is needed in order to formulate specific advice. We still do not know the actual relevance of the various proposed discords.

The tribal way of living began to disappear 10,000 years ago with the advent of agriculture. Social relations within the community have changed dramatically since then. The lack of a tribal setting may, in fact, be the most significant discord between present life and that of the human EEA. Without our strong, innate social propensities, large-scale societies would never exist. And yet, due to the difficulties of avoiding social discords, human interactions may prove to be an Achilles heel for the human species.

In industrialised countries there are numerous mismatches associated with how we evolved to interact with other individuals. For example, the close-knit tribal world of the Palaeolithic era has been replaced with nuclear families, and a relatively weak and unstable social network. In the tribal world, there was always someone around for comfort, and relations typically lasted for life. The culture, including morals and ways of behaviour, was stable, implying that people knew how to deal with each other as well as what to expect. Transactions were among affiliates, so the individual could trust that social contracts were heeded.

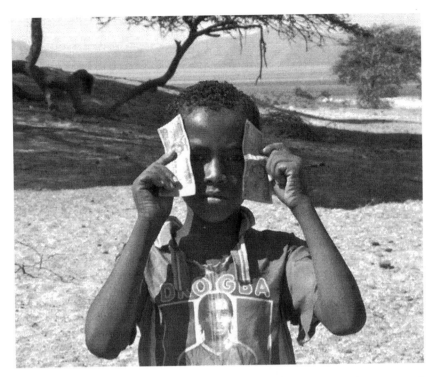

Fig. 7.2 Does money buys happiness? This Ethiopian boy may think so, but the experts are in doubt. In fact, money may act as blinkers shielding both individuals and governments from seeing what really matters as to quality of life. (Photo: B. Grinde)

Today, most people experience daily encounters with strangers and we are forced to deal with a range of people with whom we do not have personal relationships and who we may never meet again.

Some mismatches may not matter, or actually offer advantages, while others prove to be discords. It is, however, difficult to distinguish between mismatches and discords. Some aspects of modern living may be sensed as an advantage, but still have a negative long-term effect on the psyche. A possible example is the feeling of 'freedom' associated with not having any close ties or commitments. At the moment, we tend to prefer the liberty to do what we want, but if the long-term consequence is loneliness—due to lack of friends—the freedom may cause a reduction in happiness as integrated over a lifetime.

As argued in Chapter 6, the ambition of politics ought to be to promote well-being rather than wealth. It appears as if money tends to restrict, or distort, people's vision (Fig. 7.2). Our attention and ambitions are directed at obtaining ever more money, and/or the products to be purchased with money. The result is more likely to be overindulgence and related behaviour expected to reduce, rather than improve, lifetime happiness.

The focus on wealth can be explained as a consequence of human nature, but it may still be possible to alter our inclination towards greed and consumption. Bhutan appears to have had some success, and other nations may follow. Moving from gross national product to gross national happiness implies a lot more than simply down-playing the role of money.

It should be possible to raise the level of happiness beyond what might be expected to be the typical state based on our evolutionary history. That is, evolution designed for survival and procreation, but we can take advantage of features that bevolution has added to our brain, and opt for maximisation of happiness instead. The key elements in this pursuit are:

1. Create an environment that caters to the human psyche by avoiding discords.
2. Make sure there is sufficient incentive for production and invention in order to supply people with the necessities of life, and with state-of-the-art medical treatment.
3. Teach people to exercise their brain for the purpose of elevating the net output of the mood modules.

Of the three, the first is the most theoretically difficult to achieve; partly because the environment in an industrialised society can never return to the ideal, Stone Age environment; partly because we do not know what the discords are. We are confined to a 'human zoo', but we can try to improve the conditions by creating the optimal industrialised zoo.

The second is the most expensive; the limitations on a world basis are due to limited resources, and not limits in knowhow. The third is cheap, but not easily implemented. The data suggest we do have techniques that can improve happiness, but they require a dedicated effort. The human brain has an incredible capacity for learning and for being moulded by the environment. It is consequently possible to enhance happiness—as it is possible to enhance the capacity to memorise, to play chess or to perform a triple somersault.

In short, the three points above are all feasible; yet, for various reasons, difficult to achieve. I believe all the fancy products of human ingenuity—from allowing people to connect via Internet to sending a man to the moon—are the easy tasks. Understanding human nature, and acting upon our knowledge to create a world where happiness flourishes, is the real challenge.

For the typical charter tourist, the world seems ever more homogeneous—a planet where the dominant culture is that of Western consumerism. By looking around meticulously the dedicated globetrotter may, however, find 'islands' of a different nature. Some people never took part in the ups and downs of Western civilization. We refer to them as aboriginals or tribal people, and they still live more or less like our Stone Age ancestors. Even within industrialised nations there are those who turned their back to consumerism. They gathered likeminded people to create small-scale communes where togetherness, closeness to nature and meaningful lives should rule. These initiatives are typically referred to as eco-villages or intentional communities. Perhaps some of these islands can serve like seeds to sprout a new world culture (Fig. 7.3).

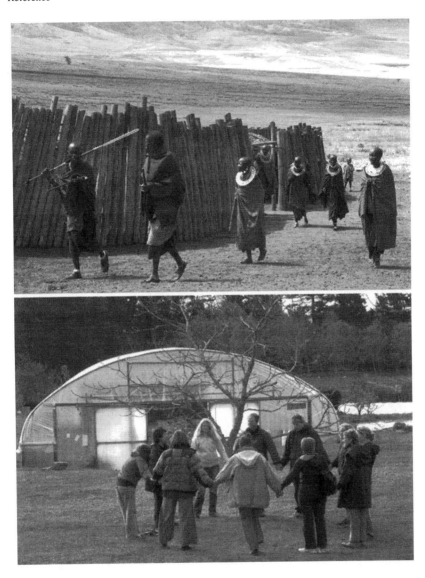

Fig. 7.3 There are places with different ideas as to how life should be lived. The Masai of Kenya and Tanzania (*above*) have kept their traditions in spite of the lure of industrialised society, and people at the ecovillage Findhorn in Scotland (*below*) are trying to re-establish some facets of tribal life in the hope of finding joy and contentment. (Photo: B. Grinde)

Reference

Panksepp, J. (1998). *Affective neruoscience*. New York: Oxford University Press.

About the Author

Bjørn Grinde received his education in Natural Sciences, Psychology and Anthropology from the University of Oslo, ending with a Dr. Scient and Dr. Philos in Biology. He is presently employed as Chief Scientist at the Division of Mental Health, Norwegian Institute of Public Health. He has previously served as scientist and professor at top universities in Norway, United States and Japan. A lasting focus has been to understand the process of evolution, particularly how it has formed the human brain and our capacity to enjoy life. He has written several books, including 'Darwinian Happiness' (The Darwin Press)—a book for a general audience that suggests how the biological perspective can be used for guidance.

B. Grinde, *The Biology of Happiness*, SpringerBriefs in Well-Being and Quality of Life Research, DOI: 10.1007/978-94-007-4393-9, © The Author(s) 2012

Made in the USA
Middletown, DE
03 May 2015